THE ULTIMATE GYM WORKOUT

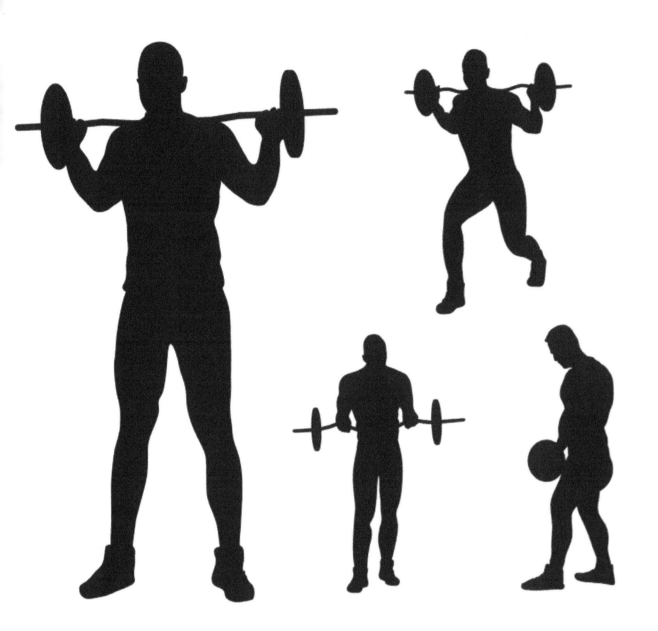

THE ULTIMATE GYM WORKOUT

YOUR DEFINITIVE GYM COMPANION

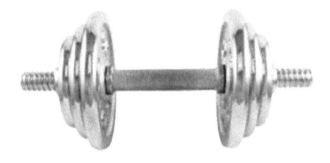

BY

DR. JONATHAN S. LEE BDS BSc

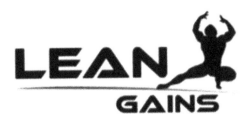

DIAMOND MEDIA PRESS CO.
1-304-273-6157
https://www.diamondmediapressco.com/

www.leangains.co.uk

Copyright © 2020

By Dr. Jonathan S. Lee

ISBN Paperback: 978-1-951302-72-6

PREFACE

My fascination with brawn began almost thirty years ago when I came across an old VHS copy of the now classic documentary 'Pumping Iron.' As I watched Arnold Schwarzenegger compete with Lou Ferrigno for the title of Mr. Olympia, my eyes were virtually glued to the screen for ninety minutes. Once it was over, the first thing I wanted to do was to grab my gym clothes, drink a protein shake (which, thanks to inspiration from the movie "Rocky," consisted of six raw eggs in a tall glass) and run as fast as I could to the local gym (which was incidentally ten miles away!). At the age of twelve, however, this would prove to be a difficult feat.

Nevertheless, I knew from that moment onwards that weight training was going to be an integral part of my life in one way or another. When I was sixteen years old, my close friend introduced me to a new gymnasium that opened up in our neighbourhood. I was finally 'old enough' to begin my weight lifting journey. Within six months, I was hooked and since then, I've never looked back. I still lift weights on a regular basis (three to five days a week) and will continue to do so for as long as I'm able.

As you can no doubt imagine, my twenty-five year love affair with weight training, food, nutrition, and exercise has consisted of many peaks and troughs. During this time, however, I've trained alongside many professional athletes, bodybuilders, power-lifters and even yoga teachers. In so doing, I was in a position to 'pick their brains' and learn about what training regime worked best for them. As time moved on, my passion for weight training and sports nutrition grew stronger and stronger, and the thought of going to university and studying these topics further became appealing to me. My dream came true in 1995 when I was accepted into King's College London. In 1999, I graduated with a Bachelor of Science Degree in Nutrition and Medical Sciences. I later studied Dentistry at Guy's Hospital, London and qualified a few years afterwards as a dental surgeon. In total, my time at university spanned eight years allowing me enough time to further my knowledge base with regards to sports nutrition, dentistry and medicine.

In the beginning of 2009, my father became very ill. A few weeks later, he was diagnosed with stomach cancer. This news came as a massive and terrifying shock to me and my family. I personally found this dark time in my life extremely difficult to come to terms with. I could not understand how such a thing could happen to someone who had led an active life, was physically strong, who'd never smoked a cigarette in his life, and rarely drank alcohol. Up until that point, my father was the spitting image of health. Ironically, my siblings and I would refer to him as 'Superman' on occasion because we'd never known him to be sick. This is why it came as an additional shock to the family when he passed away later on during that year.

illness. Then one day, whilst reading an article in a magazine, I came across an advertisement with the slogan "You are what you eat!" These five words served as a 'eureka' moment because they allowed me to concentrate less on common environmental factors that often play a role in Western diseases (such as emotional stress, pollution, smoking and so on) and shift the focus more towards dietary factors.

Despite the fact that he took pride in his physical appearance, my father did not have the best diet in the world. He would rarely eat enough fruits and vegetables, for instance, and frequently consumed foods that were either fried or heavily processed. In addition, he would exercise less frequently and start eating more 'take away' meals as he got older.

In retrospect, it is my strong belief that the combination of a poor overall diet, in conjunction with insufficient exercise, were the main reasons behind his illness and consequent demise. I also believe that if he were to apply an effective preventative nutritional approach and exercise programme as part of his daily routine, then he would still be alive today.

It is for this reason why I wrote a book entitled **'The Essential Guide to Sports Nutrition and Bodybuilding.'** My overall intention, whilst writing the book, was to not only cover the scientific fundamentals behind muscle growth and fat loss, but to also focus on the vital steps that need to be undertaken on a regular basis in order to live a long, vibrant and healthy life. My aim was to spread more awareness on the topic of disease prevention without detracting away from its relevance in the world of sports nutrition, exercise and bodybuilding. This 800-page book took over 5 years to write from its initial conception, and was finally completed and published in 2018.

I followed this up with a book called **'Lean Gains' (second edition)** which was published around the same time. In this book, I included a number of exercise routines which have been proven time and again to optimise muscle growth, increase stamina, improve fitness and accentuate fatloss.

After receiving excellent feedback from trainees, personal trainers and regular gym-attenders who undertook these exercise regimes, I decided to write this book.

As the name suggests, **'The Ultimate Gym Workout'** is a book that you can conveniently refer back to during your workouts.

The routines in this book have been carefully thought-out and designed to not only ensure that your workouts are effective, but to also eliminate any unnecessary dilly-dallying in the gym.

This book provides you with a step-by-step guide to all the exercise routines you need to undertake in order to achieve the results you've been waiting for. In addition, you will get an in-depth explanation and demonstration (ebook version) on how to do these exercises properly.

'The Ultimate Gym Workout' should be used as an adjunct to either **'Lean Gains' (second edition)** or **'The Essential Guide to Sports Nutrition and Bodybuilding.'**

I really cannot stress this enough. The purpose of 'The Ultimate Gym Workout' is to help you make the most of your workouts and (to some degree) diet. The science and reasoning behind it are intentionally left out of this book, but are covered in immense detail in my other two books.

'How To Get The Perfect Body' was my penultimate book providing an in-depth summary of the things to look out for if your main focus is to burn fat, build muscle, and to look (and feel) great.

'Lean Meals for Everyone' is my most recent book. I felt that this book was the missing ingredient (pardon the pun) to the **'Lean Gains' Book Collection.**

Eating regimes and dieting habits vary massively from one person to the next. Some dieters, for instance, would prefer a ketogenic approach, whilst others may prefer to go vegan. Many trainees prefer eating 6 small meals a day, whilst others feel more comfortable fasting for prolonged periods of time. The point is that a few random meal plans here and there is unlikely to cater for everyone. **'Lean Meals for Everyone'** contains something for everyone!

For more information about the
'Lean Gains Book Collection,'
then please visit www.leangains.co.uk

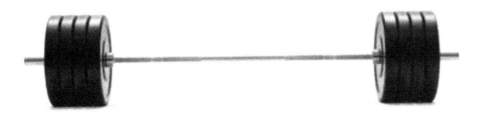

ACKNOWLEDGEMENTS

I would like to take this opportunity to thank each and every one of my mentors. They have provided me with a deep understanding of the science behind all aspects of sports-related nutrition and physiology over the last 25+ years.

I'd like to give special thanks to Dr Anthony Leeds, at Kings College London, and Professor Thomas Sanders. Their knowledge and wisdom so clearly displayed during our one-to-one tuition sessions over the years have contributed massively towards the backbone of many topics covered throughout this book.

I would also like to acknowledge the extensive research undertaken by the plethora of doctors, scientists, nutritionists and researchers whose work has been referenced throughout this book. Without their notable contribution towards the world of sports nutrition and bodybuilding, I would not have been able to undertake this project.

I wish to extend my thanks to the many personal trainers, bodybuilders, and athletes I've had the pleasure to work with. My sincere appreciation extends further to Dermot Gallagher, Jamie and Lindsey from EDC Lifestyle, Narrinder, Scott (from 'Simply Gym'), Chris Halgreen, Jayroy Buffong, and Dave "Bulldog" Beattie. Over the years, these individuals have demonstrated a superb knowledge base which has served to inspire me both inside the gym as well as throughout my daily life. I'd also like to thank these individuals for the use of 'Genesis Gym,' 'Simply Gym (Walsall), and 'Solihull College Gym' where many of the photos within the book were taken.

Finally, I wish to thank my mother and my brother for their continual love and support whilst writing this book.

CONTENTS

PART ONE : THE METHOD BEHIND THE MADNESS

PART TWO : THE GYM WORKOUTS EXPLAINED

CONTENTS

CONTENTS

CONTENTS

CONTENTS

CONTENTS

PART THREE : YOUR NEW GYM WORKOUT

PART FOUR : SOME FREQUENTLY ASKED QUESTIONS

THE 'LEAN GAINS' BOOK COLLECTION

A HANDFUL OF TESTIMONIALS

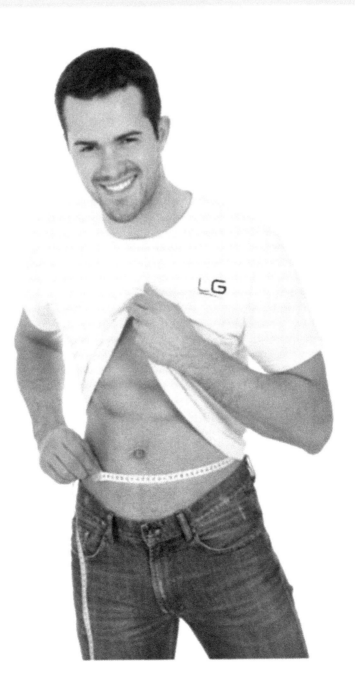

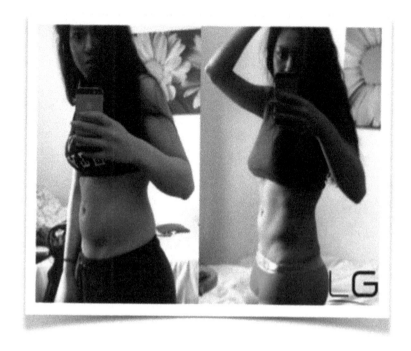

"I am so happy with these results! I've struggled in the past with weight-loss plateaus, but have finally reached may goals!"

SARAH

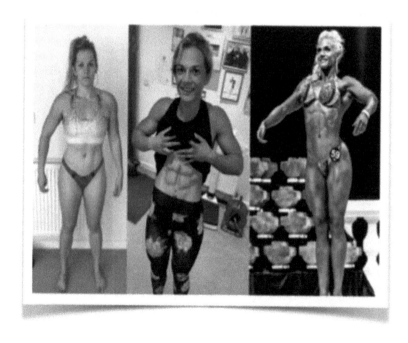

"As a female bodybuilder, I can say that "Your Pocket-book Guide to The Ultimate Gym Workout" is the perfect adjunct for those serious about making some lean gains.!"

SIAN

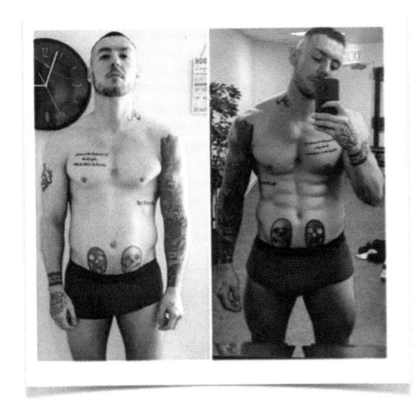

*"Speaking as a profession-
al personal trainer, I can
say that the advice in Dr
Lee's books are spot on!"*

JAMIE

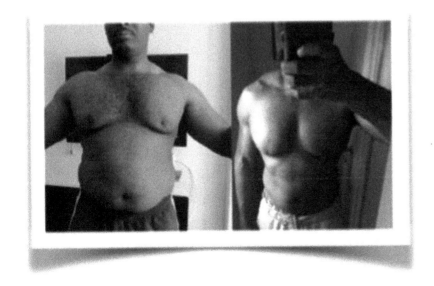

*"The routines in this book
enabled me to loose 10%
bodyfat in 10 weeks!
Strongly recommended"*

JOHN

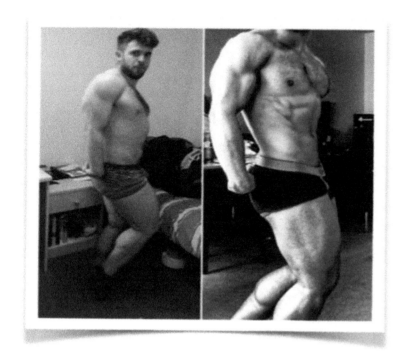

"The training and dieting regimes highlighted throughout this book are essential for success.."

CHRIS

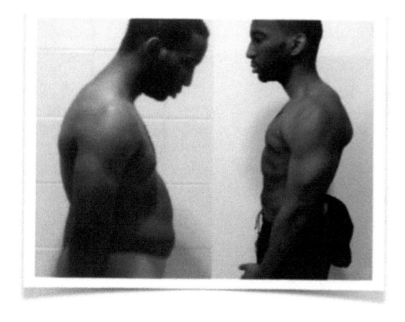

"I lost 8 pounds in 6 weeks and am more than happy with the results. Everything I did to get there is explained in this book!"

MICHAEL

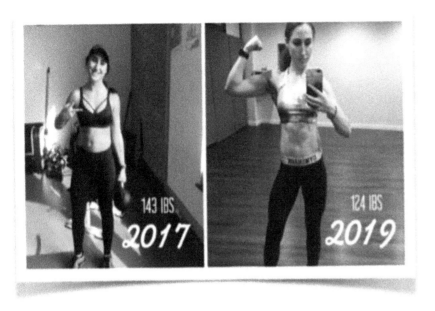

"'The Ultimate Gym Workout' is an absolute must for those looking to make some 'lean gains!'"

MOLLY

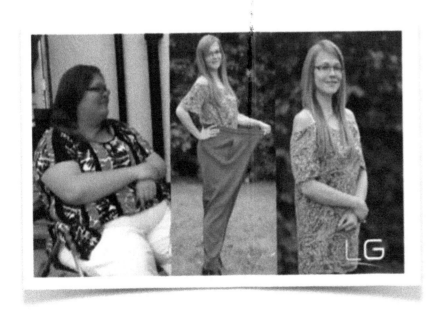

"I was over 21 stone, and I lost 12 stone in weight in under 2 years. The nutritional advice and dieting regimes in all of Dr. Lee's books are spot on! "

MICHELLE

ABOUT THE AUTHOR

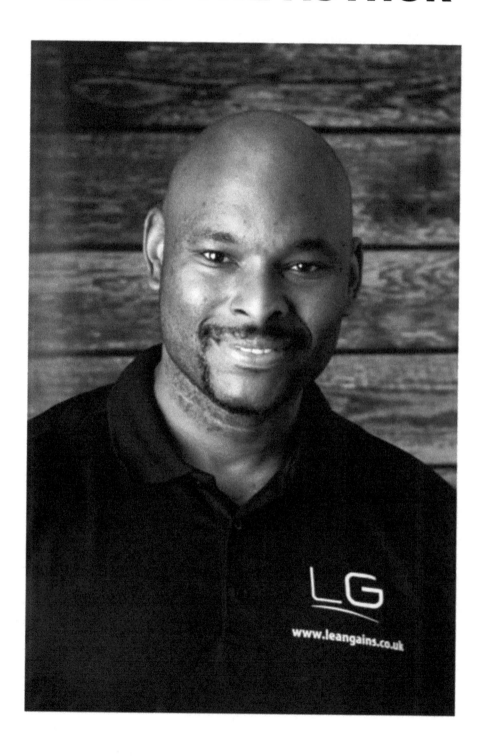

DR JONATHAN S. LEE.....

...is a **qualified sports nutritionist and personal trainer** who has successfully worked with thousands of clients over the past 20 years.

In his early twenties, **Dr Lee was clinically obese** with a body fat percentage of 28. He struggled with obesity for over 3 years trying out a multitude of diets and 'get ripped quick' fitness regimes.

When these fad diets and fitness programmes inevitably failed, Dr Lee made the wise decision to study this topic in more detail by going to university. He graduated from **King's College London in 1998 with a Bachelor of Science in Nutrition and Medical Science.**

He spent the next 5 years of his life researching the science behind fatloss, muscle growth, healthy living, fitness, and weight training.

In the meantime, he was able to burn **18% body fat in only 10 months!!** This incredible achievement was a strong enough incentive to become a personal trainer in 1999 to help other people reach their fitness goals.

He wrote his first book 'Lean Gains' in 2016 and has since written **6 more health and fitness book**

For more information,
visit www.leangains.co.uk

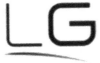

ABOUT THE BOOK

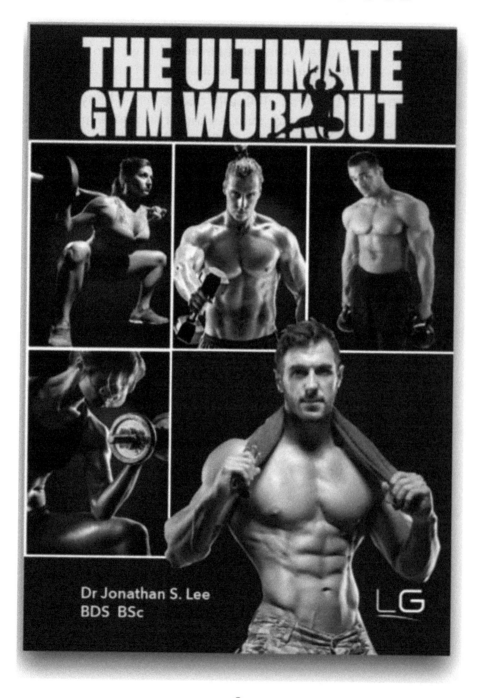

WHAT WILL <u>YOU</u> GET
OUT OF THIS BOOK?

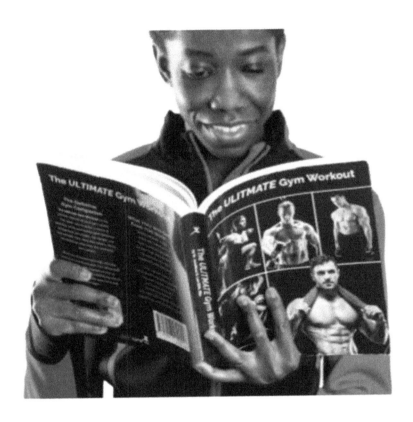

This is the **fourth** book in the **'Lean Gains'** series, and is probably the **most relevant** when it comes to providing gym-goers, dieters, and bodybuilders with direct, 'over-the-shoulder' training advice (both inside and outside of the gym)…

……WHAT THE HELL ARE TALKING ABOUT JON???!!…. …

Good question….

….Uhr, Okay. Well put it this way…

...IF YOU'RE....

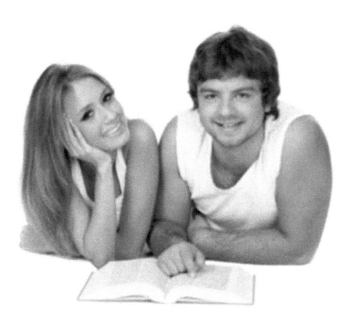

• looking for a simple yet very effective training regime that **will** get you the results you've always wanted.

• Intimidated by the million and one machines you willingly avoid each and every time you go to the gym.

• Not doing the exercises properly (i.e., with adequate form, posture, etc.) but are too embarrassed or shy to ask for help.

• Sick of paying some personal trainer for hour-long sessions, only to completely forget everything he/she told you by the following week.

• Looking for simple, no-BS diet and nutritional advice?...

......THEN CONGRATULATIONS!!.....
THIS BOOK IS <u>DEFINITELY</u> FOR YOU!!!!

......SO, LET'S GET STARTED!!!!

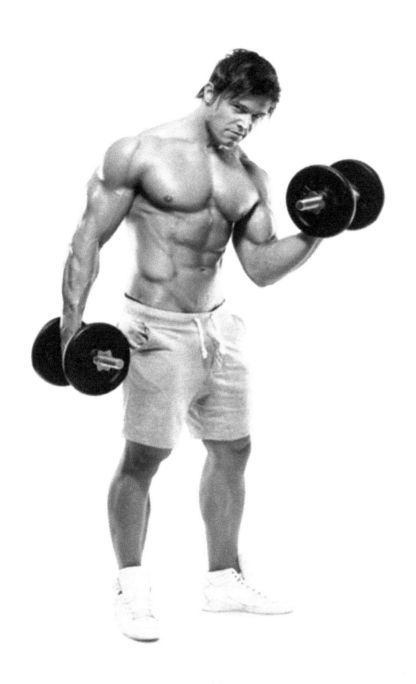

PART ONE

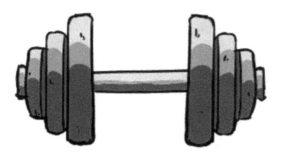

THE **METHOD**
BEHIND
THE **MADNESS**

WHY BOTHER GOING TO THE GYM?

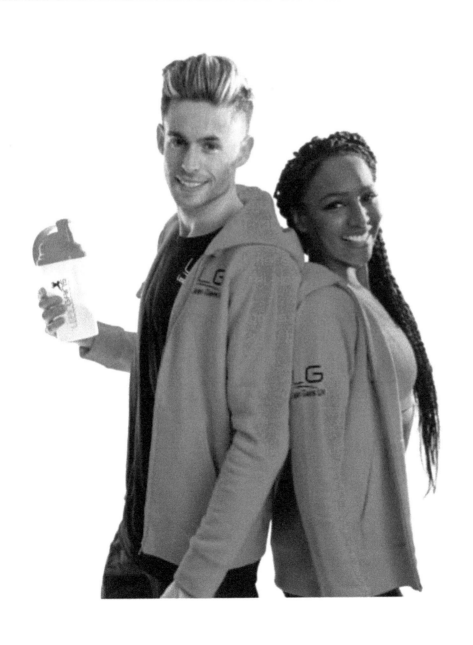

HERE ARE JUST <u>10 REASONS</u>
WHY WE SHOULD GO TO THE GYM

1. <u>MAINTAIN AND GAIN MUSCLE</u>

The aim of our workouts, especially when it comes to weight training, is to maximise muscle growth whilst bulking and minimise muscle loss during a cut.

We do this by ***progressively increasing*** the weight or number of reps as time goes on.

This is known as **'Progressive Overload.'**
Another popular way of growing/maintaining muscle is through something called
'Time-Under-Tension (TUT).'

'TUT' is the length of time that the muscle is under stress.

This takes place when you elongate the muscle by slowly releasing the weight to its original position.

2. <u>BURN OFF THAT UNSIGHTLY FAT</u>

You're going to find it more difficult to burn fat in the long-term if you're not training.

If you're not giving your muscles a good workout on a regular basis, they will shrink!!…***That's not good!!***

The combination of lean muscle in addition to a regular exercise routine will boost your metabolic rate.

This basically means that not only will you be burning a ton of calories in the gym, but you'll also be burning fat when you're sitting at home watching **Netflix**, which is an additional bonus!

3. GAIN STRENGTH

This is especially the case when you apply 'progressive overload' to your weight training sessions.

In other words, the more you lift,
the stronger you'll become.

This doesn't just apply to your muscles neither. You'll also get stronger bones as well which can reduce risk of developing osteoporosis later on.

4. IMPROVE INSULIN SENSITIVITY

We want to attain and maintain insulin sensitivity whether we're bulking or cutting.

A **high-insulin sensitivity** increases the chance of muscles utilising calories from food as opposed to these calories being stored as fat.

5.IMPROVE BALANCE

When you lift weights, you will develop a better mind-
muscle connection with time.

This improves your coordination and balance both inside
and outside of the gym.

6.IMPROVE PHYSICAL APPEARANCE

Weight training and cardio on a regular basis will not only **increase
muscle gain and fat loss**, but will also **improve skin tone**.

Your skin will naturally become more elastic, smooth and supple as
a direct consequence of training regularly.

7.HEALTH BENEFITS

Over the age of 30, most people start to lose approximately 3-8%
of their muscle per decade.

This is a condition known as **sarcopenia**.

Sarcopenia comes with a whole host of problems including
diabetes, weight gain, dementia, depression, and the list goes
on. The good news is that weight training can prevent and even
reverse this.

8. IMPROVE BRAIN FUNCTION AND MEMORY

Regular exercise increases blood flow to the brain and improves cognitive ability.

This means that exercise, especially weight training, can help you remember and focus on things much better.

9. BOOSTS CONFIDENCE

Your confidence will go through the roof once you start a well-designed weight training programme.

This will become apparent both inside and outside the gym.

10. IMPROVES MOOD

Once you start going to the gym on a regular basis, you will start to feel good. This is largely due to the release of 'happy hormones' such as **dopamine, serotonin, and endorphins**.

You produce these hormones in abundance after exercise, and more so after weight training and high intensity exercise.

DESIGNING AN EFFECTIVE PROGRAMME

An effective and sustainable gym routine has to **embrace weight training**, whereby the long-term focus revolves around *progressive overload* and *time-under-tension*.

You should also include some cardiovascular exercise (or cardio) into your routine.

It is paramount, however, to undergo a thorough warm-up beforehand, irrespective of your workout, in order to get the muscles ready for the gruelling session ahead. Failure to warm up properly can (and often does) lead to injury.

….Oh, and one more thing you can add to the list. A touch of muscle confusion. Muscle confusion revolves around the idea of growing muscle by changing your workouts every so often.

The truth is that there's **very little evidence** to suggest that regularly changing your workout regime is any better than applying tried-and tested methods such as progressive overload to your routine.

However, it does have its place, especially when it comes to directly (or indirectly) working out smaller muscles that are sometimes neglected.

BABY STEPS ARE EVERYTHING!!!!

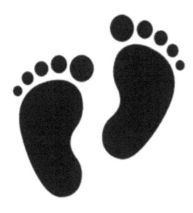

The best way to achieve success in any and
every endeavour **we** do in life is to:

1) Plan what you're doing in advance,

2) Remain focussed and consistent,

3) Gradually progress and improve.

The same is true when it comes to the gym.

This is why it's paramount that you apply these principles to your workouts.

The following page shows examples of how you can apply progressive
overload and take baby steps to gradually improve your performance in the
gym.

WEIGHT TRAINING EXAMPLES

Aim: To Get A Bigger ChestĀ

Week 1: Bench Press, 6 reps, 80kgĀ

Week 3: Bench Press, 8 reps, 80kgĀ

Week 5: Bench Press, 6 reps, 84kgĀ

Week 8: Bench Press, 8 reps, 84kgĀ

Week 10: Bench Press, 6 reps, 86kgĀ

Aim: To Get Bigger LegsĀ

Week 1: Squats, 6 reps, 80kgĀ

Week 3: Squats, 8 reps, 80kgĀ

Week 5: Squats, 6 reps, 84kgĀ

Week 8: Squats, 8 reps, 84kgĀ

Week 10: Squats, 6 reps, 86kgĀ

The Bottom Line

The actual numbers used in the above examples are arbitrary. The point is to slowly increase the number of reps and weight over time. By doing this, your muscles will slowly grow bigger.

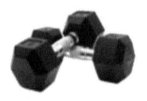

CARDIO EXAMPLES

Aim: <u>To Burn Off More Calories</u>

Week 1: Walking, 10 minutes, 2 days/week

Week 2: Walking, 15 minutes 2 days/week

Week 3: Walking, 20 minutes 2 days/week

Week 8: Jogging, 10 minutes 2 days/week

Week 10: Jogging, 15 minutes 2 days/week

Aim: <u>To Burn Off More Calories</u>

Week 1: Slow Cycling, 10 minutes 2 days/week

Week 2: Slow Cycling, 15 minutes 2 days/week

Week 3: Slow Cycling, 20 minutes 3 days/week

Week 6: Faster Cycling, 10 minutes 2 days/week

Week 8: Faster Cycling, 15 minutes 2 days/week

Week 10: Fast Cycling, 15 minutes 2 days/week

<u>The Bottom Line</u>

The actual numbers used in the above examples are arbitrary. The point is to slowly increase the duration and/or intensity on a gradual basis over time.

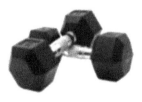

DIET: BURNING FAT

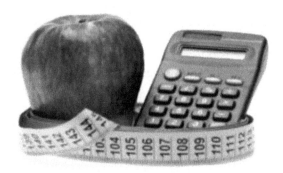

Aim: <u>Burn The Fat, Keep The Muscle</u>

1. Calculate Maintenance Calories
2. Reduce Calorie Intake by 15%
3. Consume Enough Protein = 1g/pound
4. Consume Enough Fat = 0.3-0.5g/pound
5. Consume Enough Fibre = 30g/day
6. Remaining Calories Come From Carbohydrates.

The 'Lean Gains' Book Collection

The aim of this book is to focus on **workout regimes, exercise and ntness.** Diet and nutrition is covered in <u>immense</u> detail in my other books. To learn more about your new diet regime, then please check out my other books, **'Lean Gains (2nd Edition), 'The Essential Guide to Sports Nutrition and Bodybuilding,' or 'How to Get The Perfect Body.'**

DIET: BUILDING MUSCLE

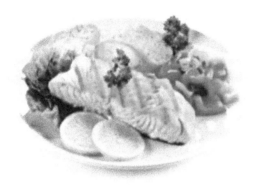

Aim: <u>Build New Muscle with Minimal Fat Gain</u>

1. Calculate Maintenance Calories
2. Increase Calorie Intake by 10%
3. Consume Enough Protein = 1g/pound
4. Consume Enough Fat = 0.3-0.5g/pound
5. Consume Enough Fibre = 30g/day
6. Remaining Calories Come From Carbohydrates.

The 'Lean Gains' Book Collection

The aim of this book is to focus on **workout regimes, exercise and ntness**. Diet and nutrition is covered in <u>immense</u> detail in my other books. To learn more about your new diet regime, then please check out my other books, **'Lean Gains (2nd Edition), 'The Essential Guide to Sports Nutrition and Bodybuilding,' or 'How to Get The Perfect Body.'**

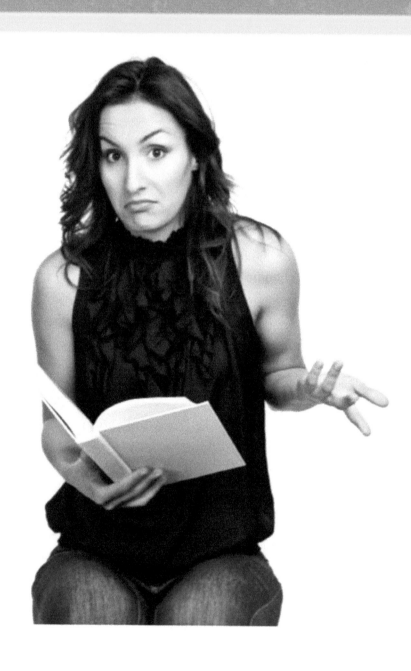

SOME FANCY JARGON
YOU NEED TO KNOW

TERMINOLOGY YOU NEED TO BE AWARE OF

1. BARBELL

Barbells are long, straight metal bars with sleeves
on the ends to hold weight plates.

There are many different barbells (16 types in total) but the **two commonest types** of straight barbells are **standard** and **olympic**.

There are 2 Olympic Bars. The Male olympic bar is heavier than the female olympic bar, but both are commonly found in commercial gymnasiums.

FEATURES	MEN'S OLYMPIC BAR	WOMEN'S OLYMPIC BAR	STANDARD
Length	7ft	6.6ft	5-6ft
Weight	20kg	15kg	7-11kg
Diameter (Grip Section)	28mm	25mm	25-28mm
Use	Found in most commercial gyms	Found in most commercial gyms	Often used in home gyms
How Much Weight It Can Carrry	360-454kg	360-454kg	70-150kg

Barbells allow you to lift heavier weights with more stability when compared to dumbbells and are best used for exercises such as deadlifts and squats.

2. DUMBBELL

Dumbbells are like short barbells which you can hold in one hand and they're typically 10 to 15 inches long.

Dumbbells allow a lot more flexibility when it comes to range of motion, and are frequently used for isolation exercises such as bicep curls, tricep extensions, lateral raises, etc. [will be discussed later].

3. REPETITIONS

A Rep is one complete motion of exercise. For example, one rep of bench press exercise would include lifting the weight, holding the weight at that position and then returning it to your starting position.

4. SETS

A Set is a group of consecutive reps. For instance, if you did ten reps of bench press, that would be one set. Two sets of ten means you did ten reps, had a rest and did ten reps again.

5. REST INTERVAL

A **Rest Interval** refers to the short break between sets during a training session.

6. ONE-REP MAX

- **1RM** refers to the absolute maximum amount of force that can be generated with one contraction. In other words, the highest amount of weight you can lift one time only.

- So let's say you're doing a bench press with a barbell, and the maximum amount you can lift at any one time is 100kg. Then 100kg would be your 1RM. Using the same example, 70kg for bench press would be 70% of your 1RM.

7. COMPOUND EXERCISES

Compound Exercises involve multiple joints and activate multiple muscle groups. More muscle groups are recruited and used per compound exercise than with other exercises. Examples include barbell-deadlifts, barbell-squats and barbell-benchpress.

8. ISOLATION EXERCISES

Isolation Exercises involves and activates primarily one muscle group only.

Examples include calf raises [activating calf muscles], cable fly [activating chest muscles] and dumbbell-biceps curl [activating bicep muscles].

9.   TRAINING TO FAILURE

Training to Failure basically means training and repeating an exercise until you physically can't do it anymore.

An example of training to failure would be doing biceps curls repeatedly until your muscles can no longer provide enough force or energy to do another rep no matter how hard you try.

10.   PROGRESSIVE OVERLOAD

Progressive overload involves gradually increasing the exercise demand and physical stress on your body to achieve continual improvement. By increasing the weight and/or number of reps over time, you're creating a continual stimulus for muscle growth.

Progressive overload requires a gradual increase in volume, intensity [weight], frequency or time.

11.   RECOVERY

Recovery is the return to prior baseline of performance.

For example, if on Monday, you could lift 6 sets of 10reps for 100kg benchpress, it may be harder to do the same on Tuesday. If by Thursday, your muscles have recovered, you should be able to lift the same 6 sets, 10 reps of 100kg benchpress.

12. <u>PERIODISATION</u>

- **Periodisation** is the process of dividing an annual training plan into specific time blocks. Each block has a particular goal and provides your body with different types of stress.

- The foundation of periodisation revolves around 3 cycles; the macrocycle, the mesocycle, and the microcycle.

- The overall aim is to reach the best possible outcome (in this case, muscle growth) over a long time period (one or more years).

- Periodisation revolves around four stages including endurance, intensity, volume, and recovery.

13. <u>THE MACROCYCLE</u>

- **The Macrocycle** is the longest of the 3 cycles and lasts up to 1 year. It incorporates all 4 stages of periodisation. Macrocycles give the trainee an overview of the training regime in the long-term so as to plan for optimum success.

- For instance, if your aim is to gain 20 pounds of muscle in a year, or to lose 30 pounds of body fat, then you can plan your desired weight 1 year from now. You can then work backwards to map out the micro- and mesocycles necessary to achieve your goals.

14. THE MESOCYCLE

A Mesocycle is a phase of training with a duration of between 2-6 weeks (for microcycles).

In the case of weight-lifting, a mesocycle can be defined as a number of continuous weeks whereby the training programme emphasises the same type of physical adaptions including muscle growth and anaerobic capacity [ie. how long the working muscle can work under an intense load before hitting fatigue].

15. THE MICROCYCLE

A Microcycle is a phase of training with a duration of a few days to around 4 weeks.

For instance, a 6 week mesocycle of strength training would consist of weekly microcycles whereby you're ideally lifting more each week for 6 weeks.

16. DELOADING

Deloading is a strategy used to aid recovery by significantly reducing the weight and/or volume that you're pushing/pulling. By doing this, you're allowing the muscles and the central nervous system to recover without compromising your workouts.

17. CARDIOVASCULAR EXERCISE

Cardiovascular exercise is any activity that increases heart rate and respiration (breathing rate) while using large muscle groups repetitively and rhythmically.

18. BULKING

Bulking is a term used by bodybuilders/weightlifters to increase calorie-intake with the aim of adding muscle mass. An unfortunate and common side-effect of bulking is some additional fat gain.

19. CUTTING

Cutting involves reducing calorie-intake so as to lose body fat whilst maintaining muscle mass. The aim is to make the underlying skeletal muscle more visible.

20. TIME-UNDER-TENSION

'Time-under-tension' is the length of time that muscle is under stress. In other words, the longer it takes you to perform a single rep, the greater the amount of 'time-under-tension.

21. <u>CELLULAR FATIGUE</u>

You can either lift weights really quickly or really slowly. You'll struggle to do a lot of reps if you're lifting/pushing weights slowly as opposed to quickly. The movement starts off easy, but after a while becomes unbearable. This is known as 'cellular fatigue' (similar to time-under-tension).

22. <u>WORKING SETS/MUSCLES</u>

These are the muscles directly involved in specific weight training exercises. They are usually used to describe the exercise after a sufficient warm up has been completed. For instance, a 'working set' would not include the preceding warm up sets.'

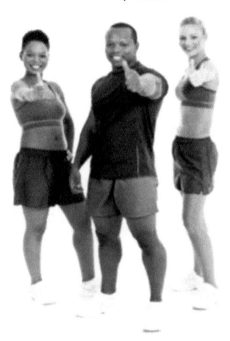

23. THE 'RATED PERCEIVED EXERTION' (RPE) SCALE

The RPE scale is used to measure the intensity of your exercise. It ranges from 0-10.

0 = Nothing at all; 10 = Very intense.

The table below highlights how RPE relates to weight training.

RPE	EXPLANATION	RPE	EXPLANATION
0	Doing nothing at all.	7	Weight used mainly for power and strength (5-7 reps)
1-4	Light weight that's used for mobility and recovery.	8	A Very Heavy Weight (allowing 2-4 reps).
5	Weight used as warm-up for heavier weight.	9	Very close to failure allowing for only 1 (more) rep.
6	Weight that can be moved quickly and performed with some speed. (eg. 8-12 rep set).	10	You've hit failure and can no longer do any-more reps.

YOUR NEW
WORKOUT REGIME

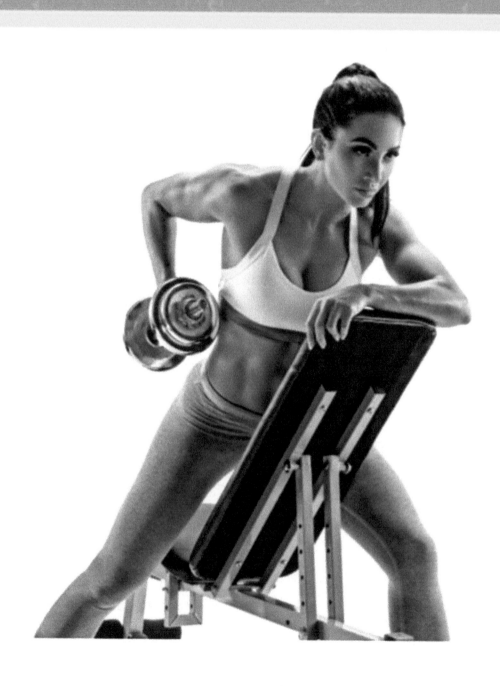

THE MUSCLES WE NEED
TO FOCUS ON

• Your NEW workout regime will consist of **weight training and cardiovascular exercise (cardio).**

• When it comes to weight training, your workouts will revolve around 8 different parts of the body:

CHEST	BICEPS
SHOULDERS	TRICEPS
LEGS & CALVES	ABS
BACK	BUTT

• There are many popular exercises out there that target muscles in these areas. However, quality is more important than quantity.

• The great thing about the workouts in this book is that they're simple yet highly effective. It really is not my aim to bombard you with a ton of exercises that won't necessarily benefit your long-term goals.

HOW WILL THIS NEW WORKOUT REGIME BENEFIT YOU?

If you go back to page 18, you'll be reminded of all the requirements necessary for an effective programme.

My aim here was to construct a tried-and-tested workout regime that not only ticks all the boxes, but is also simple and duplicatable.

At the end of the day, I wanted something that will not only guarantee predictable results, but also works to a tee.

Before **After**

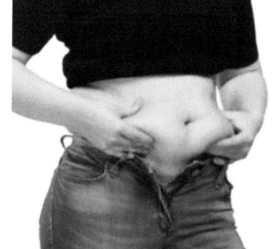
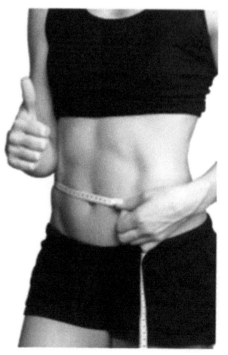

WEIGHT TRAINING

- Our principal goal is to grow and preserve muscle. This is best achieved by firstly **warming up** for 5 to 10 minutes.

- Doing this reduces risk of injury. You can then start off your main workout with the **heavy duty workouts**, usually comprising of compound exercises using relatively heavy weights.

The Essentials

Once you've **warmed up**, always start your workout with the **'essential exercises.'** The focus of the 'essential' exercises is **progressive overload.**

Do **ALL** of the 'essential' exercises in the order that they're written. Remember, the focus of the 'essential' exercises is progressive overload, so try to **add slightly more weight** each week, if possible, until you're struggling to reach the maximum rep range for that exercise.

If you can't add more weight, then focus on doing **more reps** with the same weight.

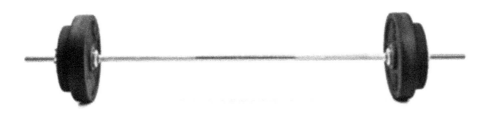

The Extras

- **Once you've done the essential exercises,** you can then choose 2 to 4 exercises of your choice from the 'extras.'

- The focus of the **'extra'** exercises is **time-under-tension and some muscle confusion.**

- You can get away with just focusing on the essentials to some degree, but the **'extra'** exercises will challenge the muscles in a different way.

- **Unlike** with the essentials, you can pick and choose up to 4 exercises to perform. Try to change these exercises every week.

- The higher rep ranges mean you can and should use lighter weights here allowing for better control of the weight. This is beneficial when you're trying to prolong the rep by focussing on time under tension.

- The choice of exercises available to you here adds diversity as well as an element of muscle confusion to the session.

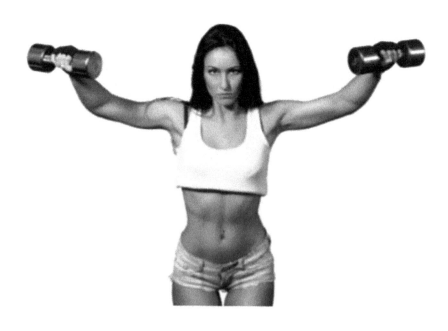

CARDIOVASCULAR EXERCISE
(Cardio)

IS CARDIO GOOD OR BAD?

Cardio is an excellent adjunct to your weight training sessions, especially if you're looking at burning off any unsightly fat.

Cardio also helps keep you fit and supple. However, doing **too much cardio**, in addition to the intense workout regimes suggested in this book, may contribute towards overtraining.

Therefore, in order to avoid overtraining, it's best to limit your cardio sessions to **no more than 3 x 45 minute cardio sessions a week on top of the workouts suggested.** This is especially the case when it comes to high intensity cardio such as sprinting, insanity-style workouts.

Also, try to do your cardio sessions at least 6 hours before or ideally after your weight training sessions to, again, avoid overtraining/burning out.

And remember what I said on page 19 about baby steps. That's very important here.

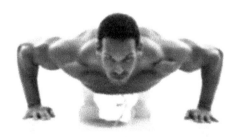

YOUR WORKOUT ROUTINE

In this section, we will give a synopsis of the
workout routines you will be doing.

They've been divided into **6 sections.**

1) BEGINNER'S WORKOUT

2) WARMING UP ROUTINES

3) OPTION A: THE 5-DAY WORKOUT

4) OPTION B: THE 3-DAY WORKOUT

5) DELOAD WEEK

6) TRACKING YOUR PROGRESS

BEGINNER'S WORKOUT

When we bear in mind the relevance of taking baby steps, it is important to keep things simple in the beginning, and progress gradually on a consistent basis.

This is why the **'beginner's workout'** must precede the more challenging workout regimes highlighted in **Options A and B.**

So, Who Is A Beginner?

A beginner is someone who either has never trained with weights before, or very rarely undertakes any weight training.

Even a regular gym-goer can be classed a beginner (or more accurately a 'de-trained weightlifter') if they have been out of the game for a while.

So, Why Are Beginners Treated Differently?

Lifting weights is crucial for maintaining muscle during fat loss and maintenance phases of your diet. Growing muscle when you're on a calorie-surplus also requires a rigorous weight training regime.

The most effective way of benefiting from weight-training in the long-term is by, therefore, setting in place a basis for our training routines.

So, why then are beginners treated differently?

Because:

• These training routines will appear foreign to the **untrained or detrained body**. A beginner should therefore not rush into a conventional strength-training programme. It's better for a beginner to adopt the necessary movements required for muscle growth.

This is why beginners should use relatively light weights for their first month or 2 whilst focussing on compound exercises. Being able to do this serves 2 purposes:

1. It provides the trainee with a foundation from which they can eventually add more weight, build muscle, and become gradually stronger whilst minimising risk of injury.

2. Using light weights from the very beginning allows the trainee to get used to training the right way, optimise their coordination, form a better mind-muscle connection, and hence undergo the required exercises with excellent form.

A workout for a beginner, using this programme, is pretty basic and essentially consists of 2 different workouts on alternate days 3 times a week.

WARMING UP ROUTINES

How Should You Warm Up?

The aim here is to gradually increase blood flow to the working muscles by making incremental increases in weight from light-to-heavy.

Warming up this way enables your body to perform at a much greater intensity when it comes to performing your working sets.

Doing a 3-5-minute light jog on a treadmill increases blood flow around the body which better prepares you for the potentially intense upcoming workout.

Once you decide which exercise you're going to do, you can follow up from this 5 minute jog with 10-12 reps at 50% of the weight you would usually lift for a set of 4-6 reps.

This works out at an RPE of around 5. You can then repeat this and then gradually increase the intensity for another set or 2 before diving into the working sets. You don't need to do more than 4 warm up sets. Remember, you need **enough energy** to perform the working sets!!!

So let's say you've just entered the gym and want to do bench press. Start off with a light jog or cycle at a gentle pace for 5 minutes. Then, if you usually lift 120kg for a set of 4-6 reps, then start off with around 60kg for10-12 reps. **This works out to be 50% intensity of your working set.**

The bottom line is that you should be lifting a weight that's very easy to move about.

Have a break for around a minute and then repeat. By this stage, you should go from **feeling cold and stiff to feeling loose and energised.**

Important Tips About Warming Up?

• **Always** do a warm-up before training each muscle group. For instance, if you're doing legs and back in one session, do a warm up for legs and then do a warm up for back once you've finished training legs.

• **Warm-up on the first exercise you're doing for each muscle group**. So if your first exercise, for instance, is military press, then warm-up on the military press [which trains your shoulders]. If you choose to move onto the next shoulder exercises, once you've completed the military press, you don't need to warm-up again. However, if you decide to train your back afterwards by doing deadlifts, for example, then warm-up on the deadlifts.

• The **'beginner's warm-up regime'** varies slightly to the other warm-ups highlighted within this book.

OPTION A: 5-DAY WORKOUT

This workout routine comprises of **five days in the gym and two days of rest**. During each workout routine, emphasis will be placed on two major muscle groups.

OPTION B: 3-DAY WORKOUT

This workout routine comprises of **three days in the gym and four days of rest**. Option B is more suited for those who prefer **not** to train five days a week. The emphasis is placed on three muscle groups per session.

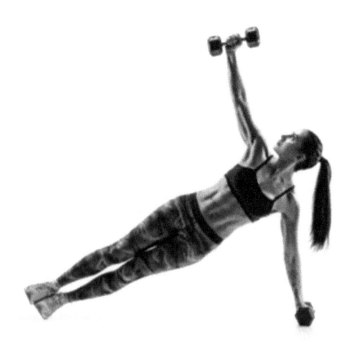

DELOAD WEEK

This **'deload' week** consists of doing easy **'beginner-style'** workouts consisting of 10-12 reps for 1 week.

These exercises are <u>intentionally</u> designed to consist of **relatively simple** and **light** workouts inflicting minimal stress to the muscles.

Lifting 'heavy' all the time creates **immense physical stress** on the body after a while, so it's essential to include a 'de-load' at the end of each training cycle [i.e., **every two months or so**] and let the body rest from strengthtraining for a while.

That way, when you're ready to go heavy again, the muscles have been well-rested and are rearing to go.

When embarking on a de-load week, ensure that you're using **relatively light weights** throughout.

The alternative to a de-load is to refrain from any weight-training at all for a week and just rest completely.

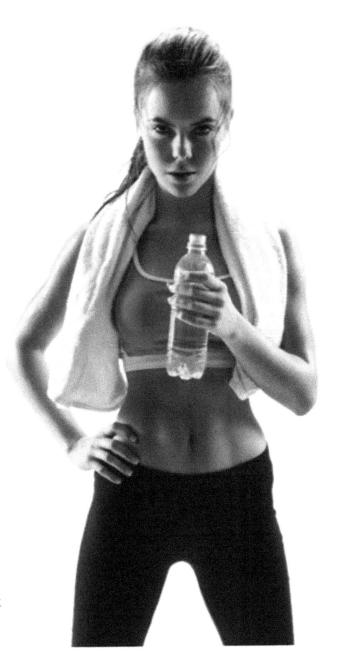

TRACKING YOUR PROGRESS

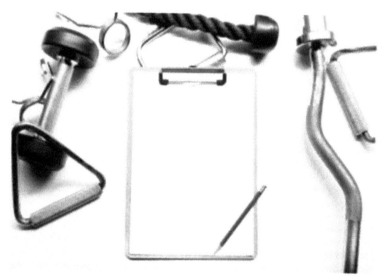

Once you get into the habits of performing the workouts in this book, your muscles will naturally become bigger and stronger over time.

Since muscle growth is a gradual progress, any gains in strength and size may not be visually apparent unless you take photos of yourself on a regular basis and document them.

The other obvious method of tracking your progress is by <u>recording and documenting your lifts.</u>

The weights you should make a note of are the ones exclusive to the working sets for the <u>essential</u> workouts only.

The prescribed workouts at the end of the book include tables which allow you to track your progress on a weekly basis.

Alternatively, feel free to download the **'Track Your Progress in The Gym'** **pdf from www.leangains.co.uk**

A FEW MORE WORDS
BEFORE WE GET STUCK IN

• The exercises and routines covered in this book are not an exhaustive list. You may come across **'new'** exercise that aren't covered here, and find them beneficial. Feel free **incorporating** a few new exercises into your regime if you so wish. However, this **does not mean** you should detract or ignore the routines outlined in this book.

• These routines are extremely effective and, in conjunction with a good dieting regime, will enable you to achieve fantastic results. By doing these exercises on a regular basis, you **will** master them.

• However, **this book is not exactly one that can fit into your back-pocket** (unless of course you're reading the e-book version on your phone).

• I **strongly suggest,** therefore, referring to the smaller version of this book entitled '**Your Pocketbook Guide to The Ultimate Gym Workout**' (available from www.leangains.co.uk). The pocketbook version is a concise book that can fit into yourback pocket. It was designed that way to act directly as a terrific aid to your workouts whilst you're in the gym.

Order your copy today from

www.leangains.co.uk

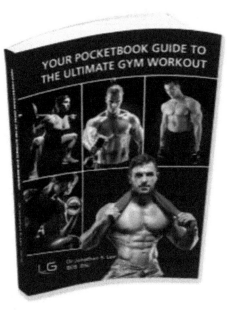

"YOUR POCKETBOOK GUIDE TO THE ULTIMATE GYM WORKOUT"

'Your Pocketbook Guide to The Ultimate Gym Workout' sets in place **tried-and-tested**, duplicatable workouts that are specifically designed to make the most of your gym sessions.

This book **fits into your back pocket**, contains **tailored 3-day and 5-day workouts** for both men and women, **cardio workouts,** and essential advice necessary to guarantee 'lean gains.'

'Your Pocketbook Guide to The Ultimate Gym Workout'
is an absolute MUST
for all gym enthusiasts.

Available from
www.leangains.co.uk

PART TWO

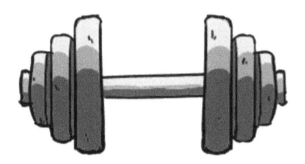

THE GYM
WORKOUTS
EXPLAINED

HOW TO PERFORM THESE WORKOUTS CORRECTLY!

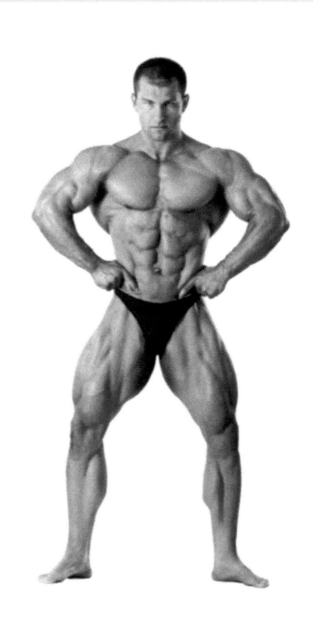

THE MUSCLES YOU SHOULD BE TRAINING

We need to take a close look into the
muscles we're training.

By doing this, we will gain a better understanding of how the
workouts in **part three** benefit the desired muscle growth.

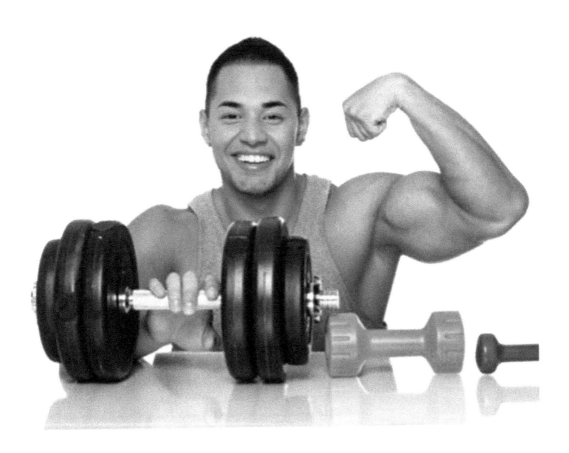

MUSCLE GROUP	EXERCISE
CHEST	BARBELL BENCH PRESS [FLAT AND INCLINED] DUMBBELL BENCH PRESS [FLAT AND INCLINED] DUMBBELL PULLOVER [UPPER CHEST] DUMBBELL FLYS CABLE CROSSOVER DIPS
SHOULDER	BARBELL MILITARY PRESS ARNOLD DUMBBELL PRESS DUMBBELL SIDE LATERAL RAISE REAR DELT RAISE [SEATED] BARBELL REAR DELT ROW DUMBELL FRONT RAISE
LEGS	BARBELL SQUAT FRONT SQUAT LEG PRESS DUMBBELL LUNGE BARBELL LUNGE ROMANIAN DEADLIFT
CALVES	STANDING CALF RAISES SEATED CALF RAISES CALF RAISES ON LEG PRESS
BICEPS	BARBELL CURL E-Z BARBELL CURL HAMMER CURL DUMBBEL CURL CHIN-UP

MUSCLE GROUP	EXERCISE
TRICEPS	CLOSE-GRIP BENCH PRESS DIPS SKULL CRUSHERS TRICEPS PUSHDOWN DUMBBELL OVERHEAD TRICEPS PRESS
BACK	BARBELL DEADLIFT WIDE-GRIP PULL-UP BARBELL ROW OBE-ARM-DUMBBELL ROW LAT PULLDOWN BARBELL SHRUG DUMBBELL SHRUG HYPEREXTENSION
ABS	CABLE CRUNCH HANGING LEG RAISES CAPTAIN'S CHAIR LEG RAISE AB ROLLER AIR BICYCLE DECLINE CRUNCH
BUTT	DEADLIFT SQUATS [WIDE AND DEEP] HIP THRUST ROMANIAN DEADLIFT BULGARIAN SPLIT SQUATS BUTT BLASTER/GLUTE MASTER
ROTATOR CUFF	FACE PULL DUMBBELL INTERNAL ROTATION DUMBBELL EXTERNAL ROTATION

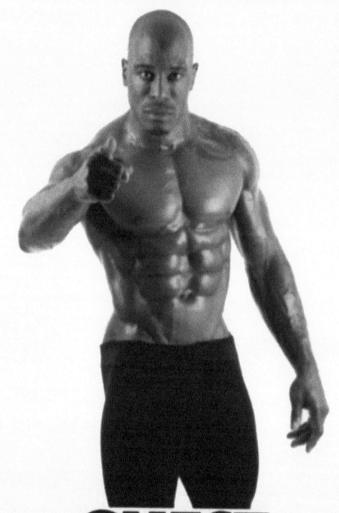

CHEST WORKOUTS

CHEST WORKOUTS

BARBELL BENCH PRESS

DUMBBELL BENCH PRESS

DUMBBELL PULLOVER

DUMBBELL FLYES

CABLE CROSSOVER

DIPS

CHEST MUSCLES

(PECTORALIS MAJOR)
THE PECTORAL MUSCLES

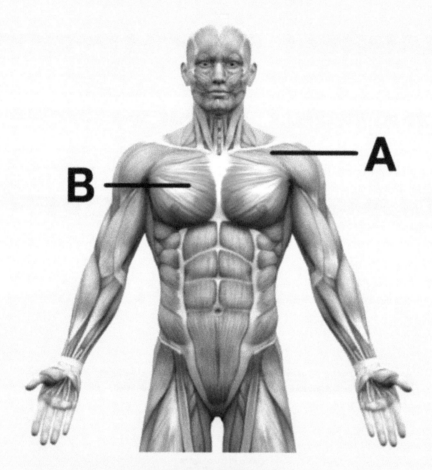

A = CLAVICULAR HEAD

B = STERNAL HEAD (MAIN CHEST)

CHEST WORKOUTS

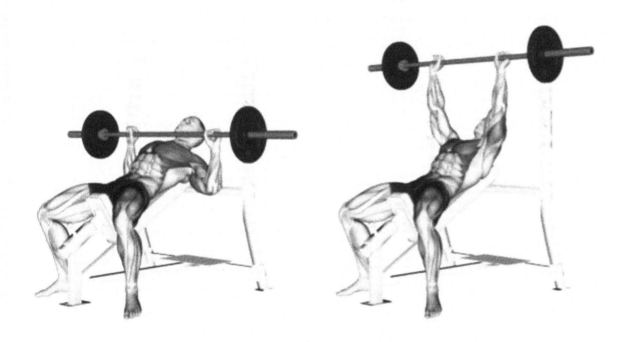

ENTIRE PECS	UPPER CHEST	LOWER CHEST
Bench Press	Inclined Bench Press	High-to-Low Cable Crossover
Dips	Dumbbell Pullover	
Dumbbell Flyes	Low-to-High Cable Crossover	

FLAT BARBELL BENCH PRESS

1. Lie Down on the bench with your **feet flat on the floor.**

2. Ensure the shoulder blades are squeezed together and down towards your waist (as if you're trying to squeeze a grape between your shoulder blades). Your grip should only be a few inches wider than shoulder width. At the same time, push your upper back into the bench.

3. **Arch your back** to maintain a neutral spine (Figure 1). It should be big enough to allow someone's fist to fit between the arch and the bench.

4. Make sure you have a firm and **tight grip of the bar**, and that you're gripping the bar as far down your palm as possible *(Figure 2)*. This is very important since if the bar is too high in your hand or fingers, you put tremendous pressure on your wrists.

5. By this stage, your body should as if it's **one firm, tight, and solid unit**. You also want to **ensure that your upper back, neck and butt are touching the bench**. At the same time your feet and heals should be flat on the floor.

6. Take a **deep breath**, stabilise your lower body by tightening your quads, abs and glutes. As you lift the bar, pretend as if you're trying to **bend the bar towards you into a U-shape with your hands.** By doing this, you're **tucking in your elbows** and hence protecting your shoulders from any potential damage.

7. As you bring the bar down, **ensure your forearms are moving up and down in a straight line** at a 90 degree angle to the floor.

8. Bring the bar down until it **touches your nipple/upper abs** *(Figure 3)*. Ensure upper arms and elbows are at around a **horizontal 45 degrees angle** to the torso when the bar is down.

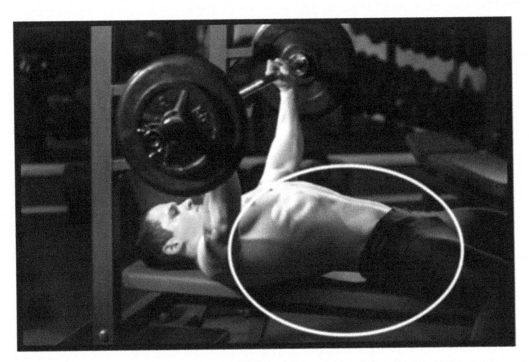

Figure 1:
Arch Your Back to Maintain a Neutral Spine.

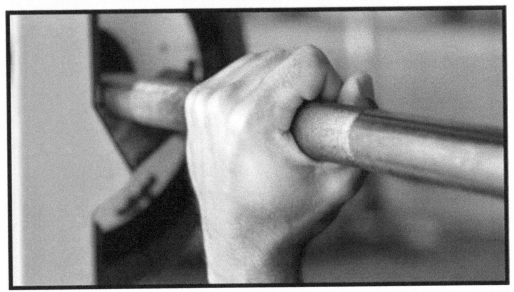

Figure 2:
Ensure that you're Gripping the Bar as
Far Down your Palm as Possible

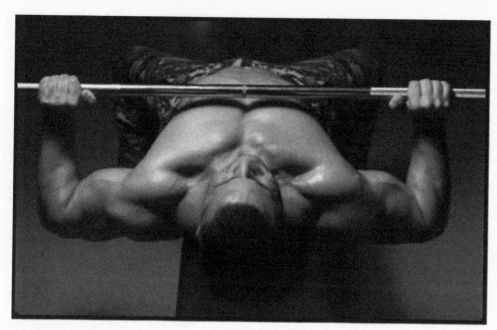

Figure 3:

Ensure bar touches your nipple/upper abs.

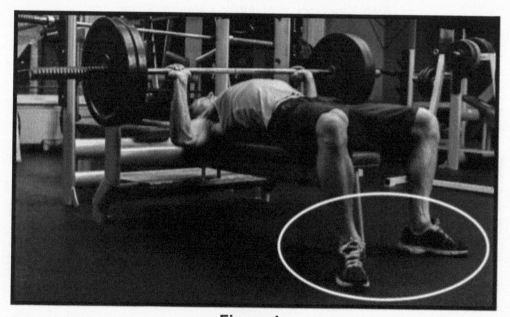

Figure 4:

Keep your feet flat on the floor throughout

the whole movement.

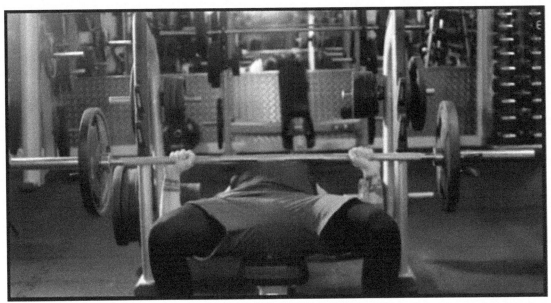

Flat Barbell Bench Press

Starting Position

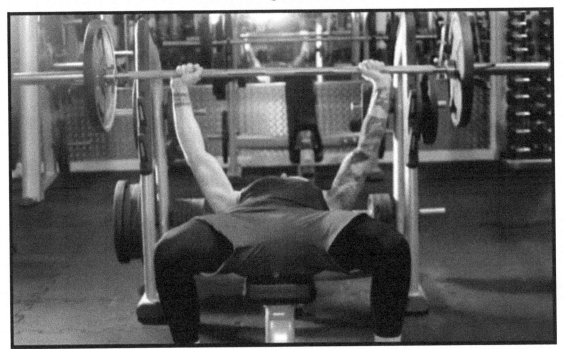

Flat Barbell Bench Press

Finishing Position

61

9. Wherever the bar touches you, **try to hit the same spot every time.**

10. **Lift the bar** by **tightening your glutes and pushing your feet into the floor** (Figure 4). This allows you to push more weight and stay tight. As you lift the bar, exhale.

11. Now unlike the squats and deadlifts (which will be discussed later on), the bar movement will **not** be a simple vertical up and down motion. Our anatomy calls for a **slight curve-path** upwards and downwards towards the rack.

Additional Tip

- Ensure a controlled and smooth motion whilst you're bringing the bar down. Do not bounce the bar off your chest. This can lead to immense stress on your shoulders and sternum.

- **Do not** flare your elbows or grip too wide as this can cause damage to your shoulders and pec muscles.

- Ensure you keep your feet flat on the floor and your core tight throughout the whole movement.

- Asking a friend to spot you is a **good idea** if you're a beginner or lifting a heavy weight.

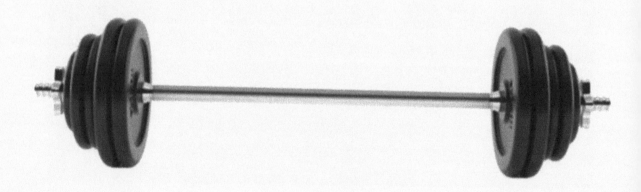

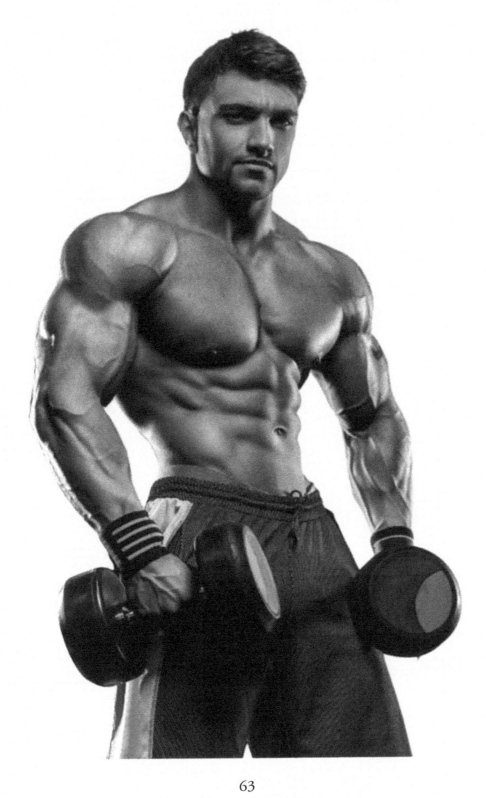

63

INCLINED-BARBELL
BENCH PRESS

- The advice is the same as for the flat barbell bench press, but:

  - Instead of using a flat bench, select a bench with a 30-45 degree angle.

  - You will be bringing the barbell down in a vertical motion passed the chin to your upper chest (just below the collar bone) as opposed to your nipple/upper torso (see Figure 5).

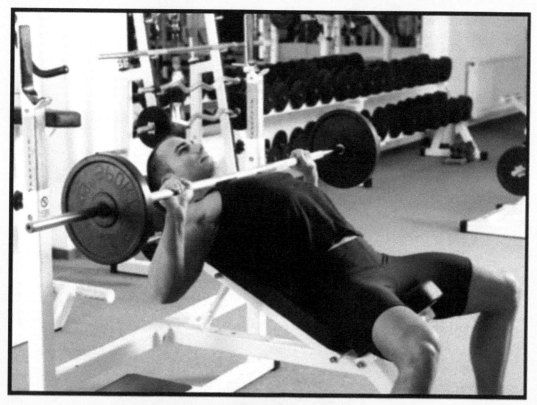

Figure 5:

Bring the Barbell Down in a Vertical Motion
Passed The Chin to Your Upper Chest.

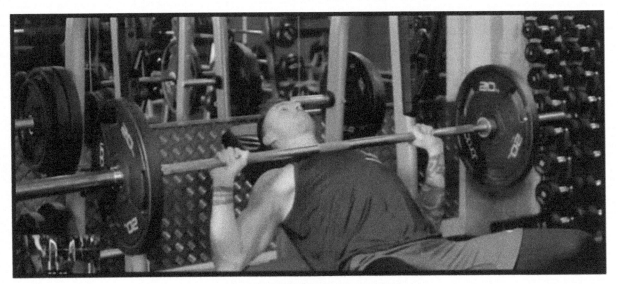

Inclined Barbell Bench Press

Starting Position

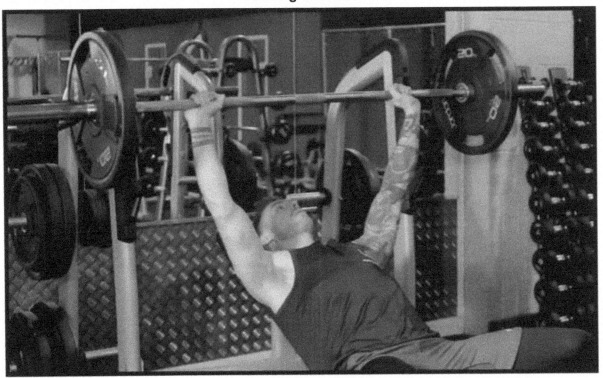

Inclined Barbell Bench

Press Finishing Position

65

FLAT DUMBBELL BENCH PRESS

- Dumbbell bench press is very similar to barbell bench press with regards to set-up, but allows for a fuller range of motion compared to the barbell bench press. This allows for a deeper stretch at the bottom of the movement and a tight contraction at the top of the movement.

- Also, because the dumbbell press requires more stability, especially around the shoulder region, you get the **additional benefit of strengthening these 'stabiliser' muscles**. In addition, if you're training to failure, **you don't need a spotter. It's much safer with dumbbells since you can simply drop the weights to the floor**.

- The only real downside with the dumbbell bench press is that you will not be able to lift as much weight as with the barbell bench press.

- So here's how you do a flat dumbbell bench press:

1. Sit down on a flat bench with your feet flat on the floor.

2. **Lean back** and bring dumbbells to shoulder level.

3. **Ensure shoulder blades are squeezed together** and down towards your waist. (Imagine trying to squeeze a grape between your shoulder blades). Your grip should only be a few inches wider than shoulder width. At the same time, push your upper back into the bench.

4. **Arch your back** to maintain a neutral spine. It should be big enough to allow someone's fist to fit between the arch and the bench.

5. Make sure you have a firm and **tight grip of the dumbbell** and rotate your wrists forward so that the palms of your hands are facing away from you.

6. Take a **deep breath at the same time as bringing your chest out**. Ensure that the dumbbells are parallel to over the lower part of your chest.

7. **Bring the dumbbells down** until just slightly wide of the outer chest. In other words, as you bring the dumbbell downwards, the inner part of the dumbbell should be just a couple of inches wide of your outer chest. You also want to make sure the dumbbells are in line with the lower part of your chest. **You don't want to hold dumbbells too wide as this will put too much pressure on your shoulder rotator cuffs which can cause damage**. This is why your shoulders should be squeezed together in the beginning. You want to use your chest to generate most of the movement; and remember to stabilise your lower body by tightening your quads, abs and glutes.

8. Ensure upper arms and elbows are at a **horizontal 45 degrees angle** to the torso when the dumbbells are in the down position. Do NOT flare your elbows.

9. **Lock your arms at the top of the movement** and squeeze your chest by bringing the dumbbells together. Hold in this position for about a second before bringing back down again.

10. As a general rule of thumb, it should take twice as long to bring the dumbbells down as it does to lift the dumbbells upwards.

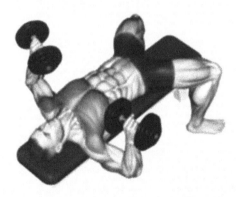

Flat Dumbbell Bench Press
Starting Position

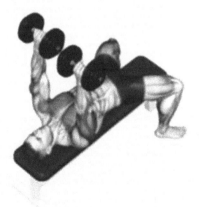

Flat Dumbbell Bench Press
Finishing Position

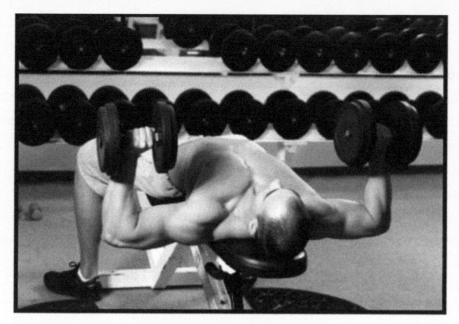

Flat Dumbbell Bench Press
Starting Position

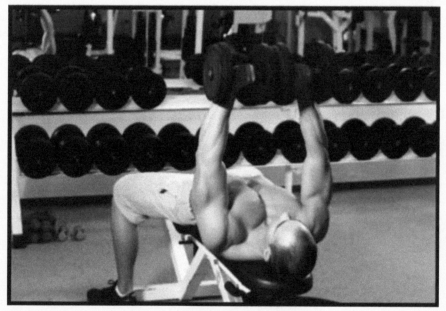

Flat Dumbbell Bench Press
Finishing Position

INCLINED DUMBBELL BENCH PRESS

- The 'inclined dumbbell bench press' exercise is very similar to the 'flat dumbbell bench press' with a few exceptions which will be discussed here.

- The bench is angled at a **30-45 degree angulation**. Bear in mind that you do have some flexibility here, but the higher the angulation, the more focus on the shoulder [deltoid] and upper pec muscles. The lower the angulation, the more emphasis that's placed on the upper and main pec muscles.

- Hold the dumbbells directly above your shoulders once the arms are fully extended. As you bring the dumbbells down, ensure they are level with the lower part of your outer chest (as with the flat dumbbell variation).

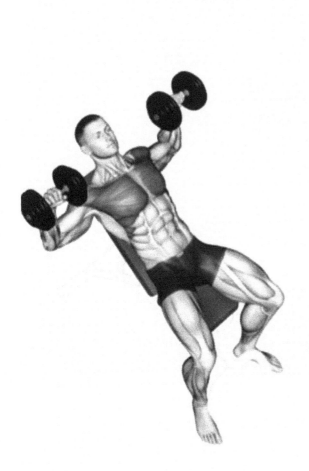 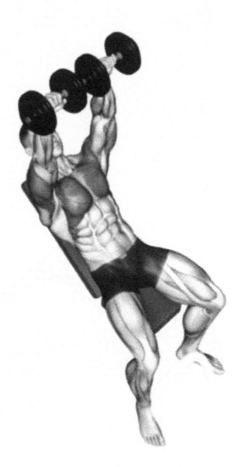

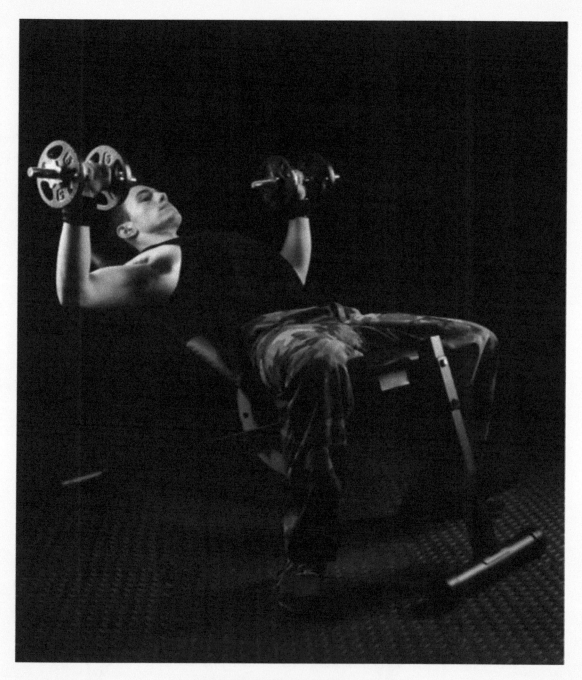

Inclined Dumbbell Bench Press
Starting Position

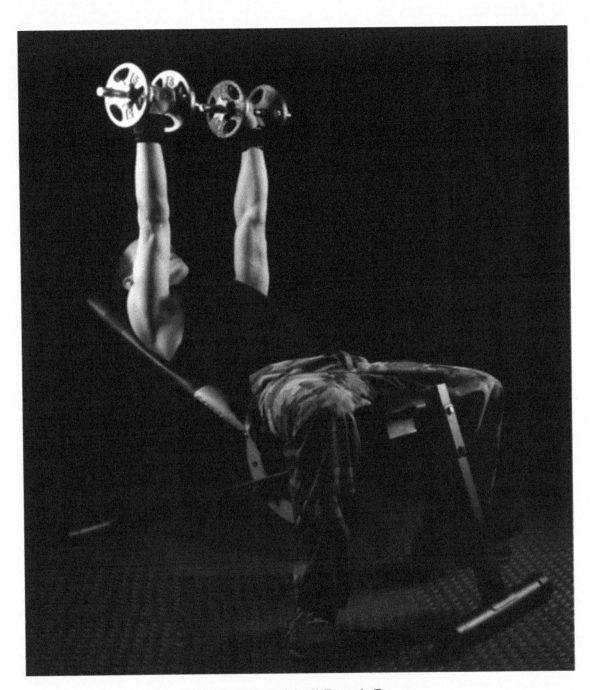

<u>Inclined Dumbbell Bench Press</u>
Finishing Position

71

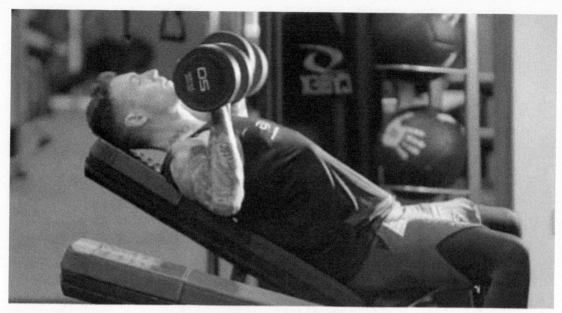

Inclined Dumbbell Bench Press
Starting Position

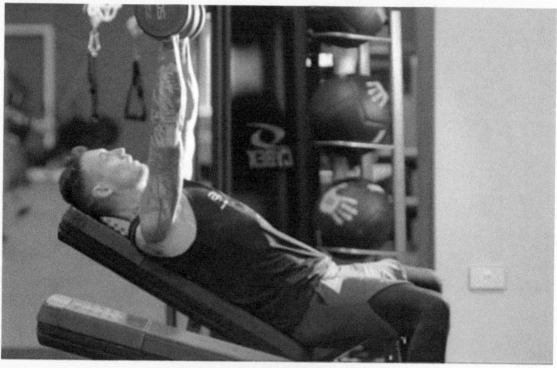

Inclined Dumbbell Bench Press
Finishing Position

A FEW WORDS OF CAUTION

- The flat and inclined dumbbell benchpress exercises are generally safe to carry out, but when you're working with heavy weights, make sure you don't descend too low. Doing so will increase the risk of damage to your shoulders (or more specifically, your rotatory cuff muscles and acromioclavicular (AC) joints).

- At the same time, you do want to feel a slight stretch in your pecs. Therefore, it's ideal to bring the weight just below the level where your elbows are parallel to the floor. However, this does not mean going to end or near end position as this will definitely cause injury (especially if you're working with heavy weights). Bring the weight only slightly below parallel until you feel a stretch (see the diagram below). Start with light weights and gradually progress to heavier weights.

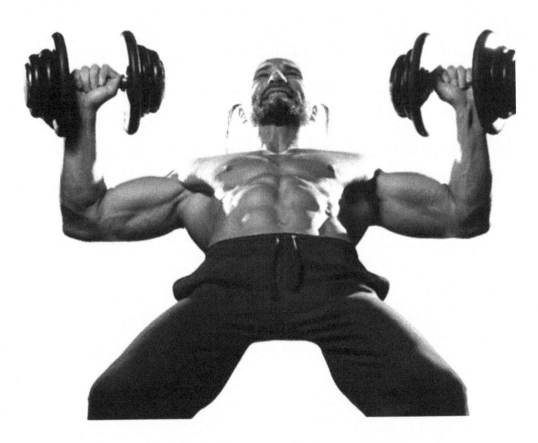

DUMBBELL PULLOVER

- There's a lot of debate as to whether the dumbbell pullover is a back exercise or a chest exercise. **In actual fact, the dumbbell pullover works out both the chest, anterior deltoids, and the upper back (lats) to some degree.**

1. Place **upper back** perpendicular to the bench and flex hips slightly.

2. Position head so it's **off the the edge** of the bench.

3. Hold a dumbbell with **both hands above your chest and with your arms fully extended**. Both palms should be pressing against the underside of one of the sides of the dumbbell.

4. Position your feet flat on the floor but spread out.

5. Keep your **hips at or slightly below the bench height.**

6. **Keep your core and glutes tight** and your arms firm with a **slight bend** in your elbow (Figure 6).

7. Retract your shoulders so that they're down and back into the bench.

8. As you bring the dumbbell backwards behind your head, **continue this movement until you feel a stretch, or almost touch the floor with the weight**. If this is too low for you, then just go down as low as you can. During this time, **keep your core tight**.

9. When you bring the dumbbell back up through this arc of motion, **ensure the core is still tight**, and bring the weight upwards until level with chest. At this point, squeeze the chest together.

Additional Tip

Keep Your Chest in an Elevated Position. This puts you in the correct position for maximum activation of the pectorals muscles.

Your chest should naturally stick up if you remember to keep your shoulders down and back, with shoulder blades squeezed together.

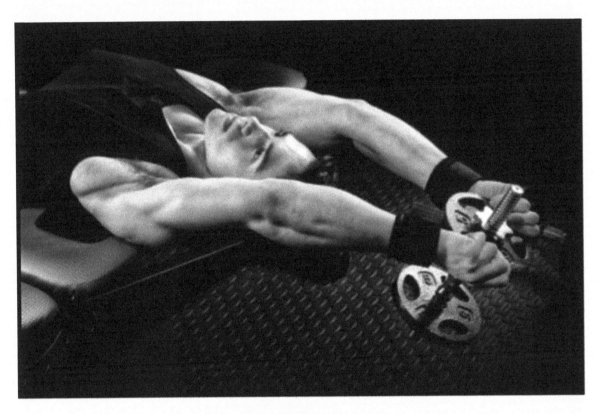

Figure 6:

*Keep A Slight Bend in Your Elbows As You Continue
The Movement Behind Your Head Towards The Floor*

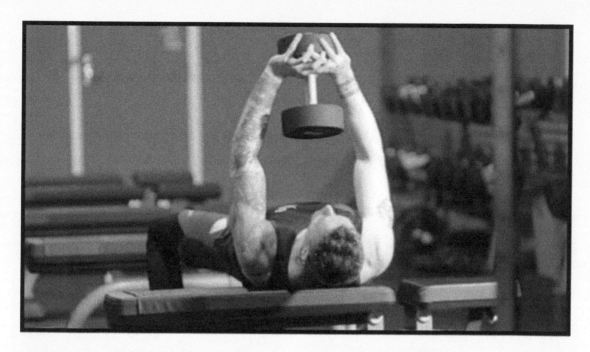

Dumbbell Pullover - Starting Position

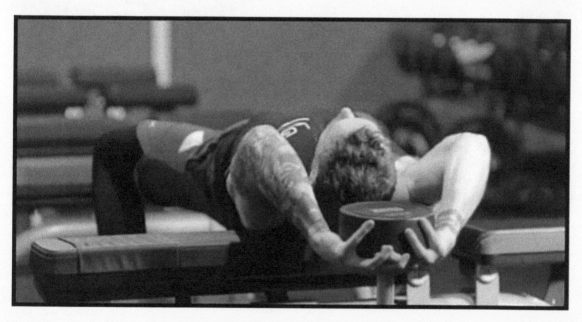

Dumbbell Pullover - Finishing Position

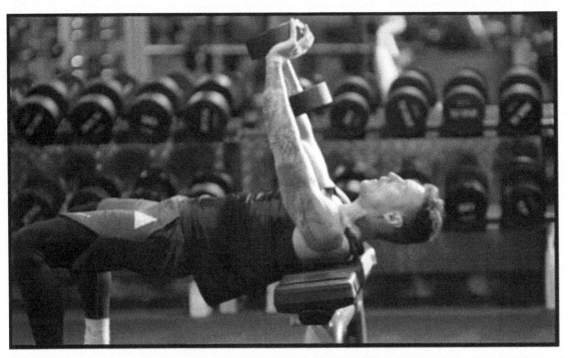

Dumbbell Pullover - Starting Position

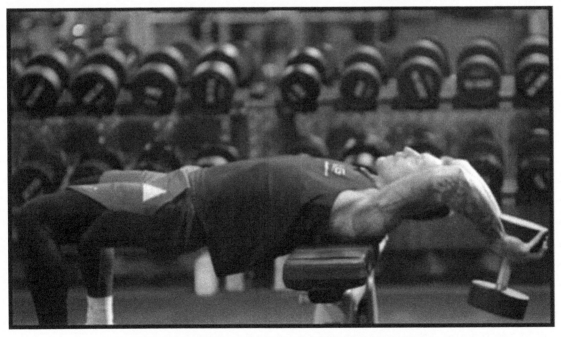

Dumbbell Pullover - Finishing Position

DUMBBELL FLYES

1. **Sit down on a flat bench** holding 2 dumbbells on your thighs.

2. Use your thighs to lift the dumbbells, lie back onto the flat bench and **hold them in front of you with palms facing.**

3. Ensure your **head and shoulders are supported by the bench** (Figure 7) and that your **feet are flat on the floor.**

4. Take a deep breath, bend your elbows slightly but hold your arms firm (Figure 8), and lower your arms at an arc until you feel a slight stretch in your chest. **Don't go any lower otherwise you run the risk of damaging your rotator cuff.**

5. Use your **pectoral muscles to reverse the movement back to the start.**

6. Return your arms back to starting position whilst **exhaling** and following the same arc of motion.

7. Hold weights together for a second whilst **squeezing your chest.**

8. Repeat.

Additional Tip

Some people go down too far on the decline movement and risk shoulder injury as a result. If you have a **pre-existing shoulder injury,** an **alternative and 'safer' version** of the 'dumbbell flyes' exercise involves following the same steps as with the conventional routine, but **not** bringing the weights lower than chest level. This way, you get to work out your chest whilst placing **minimal stress on your shoulder/rotator cuffs.**

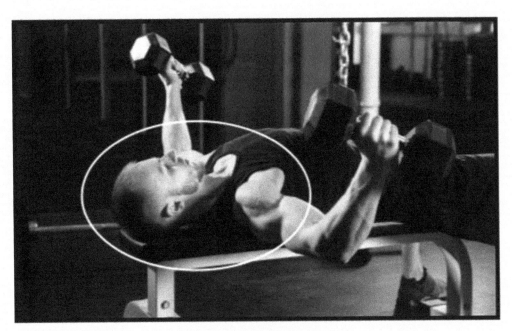

Figure 7:

Keep Your Head and Shoulders in Contact With Bench.

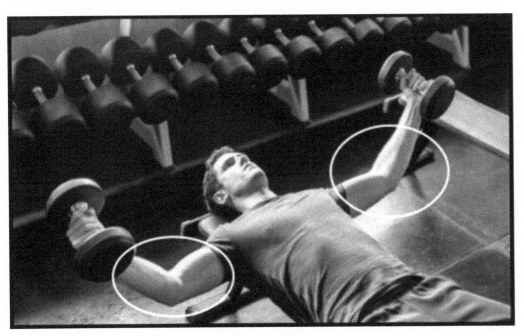

Figure 8:

Keep The Elbows Bent Slightly and Hold Arms Firm.

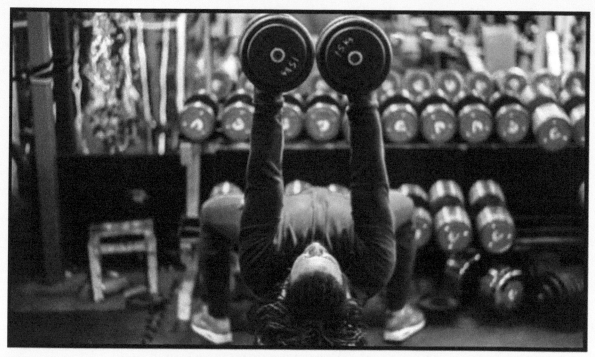

Dumbbell Flyes - Starting Position

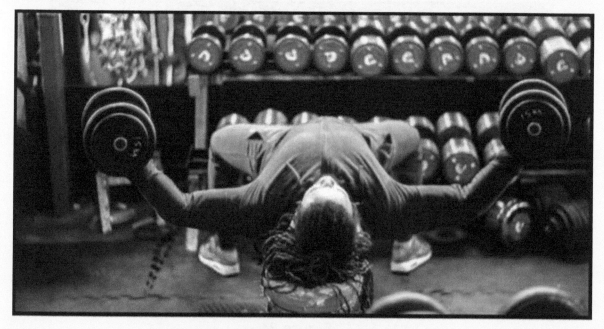

Dumbbell Flyes - Finishing Position

80

CABLE CROSSOVER

- You can use this machine to train either the lower part of the chest by moving in a downward motion (Figure 9) or upper pecs (clavicular head) by lifting the cable crossover in an upward motion (Figure 10).

LOWER PECS (STERNAL HEAD)

1. **Place pulleys on an upper position** and select the weight.

2. **Grip** the pulleys firm on each side.

3. **Step forward** as if there's an imaginary line between the pulleys.

4. Bend slightly forward but **keep your torso tight and firm.**

5. Breathe deep and bend your elbows slightly but keep your arms firm and extend them outwards until you feel a **stretch in your chest.**

6. **Bring the pulleys downwards** and towards the midline of your body.

7. Squeeze together and hold before bring pulleys back.

8. Repeat.

UPPER PECS (CLAVICULAR HEAD)

1. **Place pulleys on a lower position** and select the weight.

2. **Grip** the pulleys firm on each side.

3. **Step forward** as if there's an imaginary line between the pulleys.

4. Bend slightly forward but **keep your torso tight and firm**. Your palms should be facing forward.

5. **Bend your elbows slightly** but keep your arms firm.

6. Pull the weights/pulleys at the same time in an **upwards motion keeping your arms firm** but slightly bent at the elbows.

7. Raise the pulleys and draw your **hands upwards** towards the midline of your body. Your hands will **come together in front of your chest.** Hold and squeeze.

8. Return your hands to starting position and repeat.

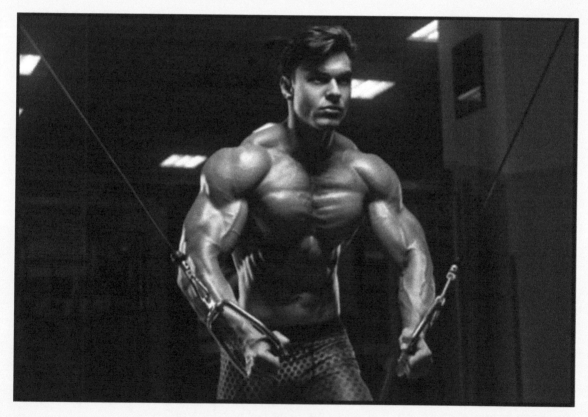

Figure 9:

Move Cable in a Downward Motion to Train Lower Chest.

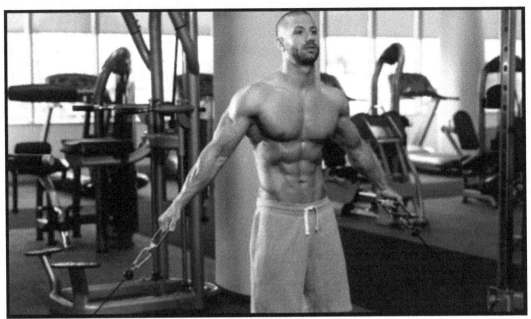

Figure 10:

Move Cable in an Upward Motion to Train Upper Chest.

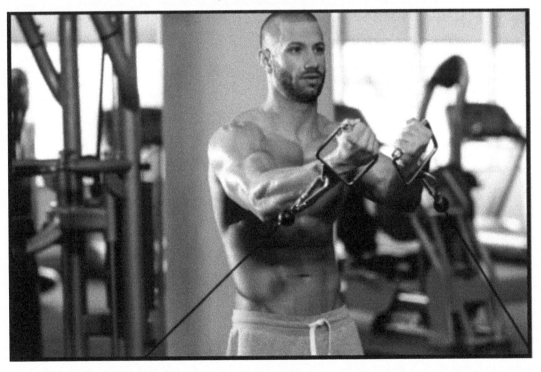

MIDDLE POSITION FOR BOTH UPPER AND LOWER PECS

A **middle/neutral** cable attachment will work
more of the mid to overall chest surface area.

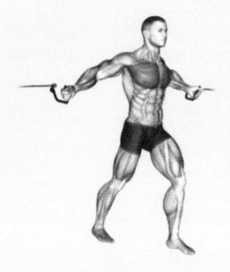

Cable Crossover - Middle/Neutral Starting Position

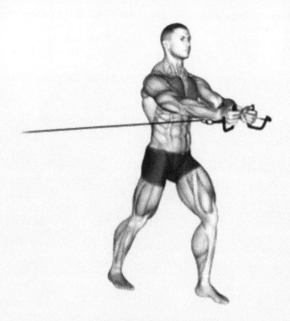

Cable Crossover - Middle/Neutral Finishing Position

DIPS

- Dips are great for both chest and triceps. However, we can position ourselves to slightly favour one over the other.

- In this variation, we are targeting the chest.

1. Grab the grip-handle hard and squeeze firmly. Your hands should be under your shoulders and just outside your hips.

2. Balance youself with straight arms and locked elbows as you enter your **start position.**

3. Raise your chest and keep your shoulders back (ie. don't roll them forward).

4. Lower your body by bending your arms and leaning forward slightly. Remember to keep your torso tight throughout.

5. Keep your legs bent and cross your feet.

6. The end position is when your shoulders are below your elbows.

7. Raise up by straightening your arms and keeping everything else firm.

8. At the top position, bring the chest outwards and straighten arms.

9. Maintain tension within the chest muscles.

10. Repeat.

<u>Variations</u>

- To exercise the pectoralis major (ie. the chest muscles), then focus more on **leaning forward when performing the dips whilst keeping the core tight.**

- **If you intend on exercising the tricep muscles, then keep your elbows close to your body whilst lowering your body.**

- **Remember** to keep your back and torso upright, and stop when there's a 90 degree angle between the upper arm and forearm. Maintain this position using your triceps to lift you up.

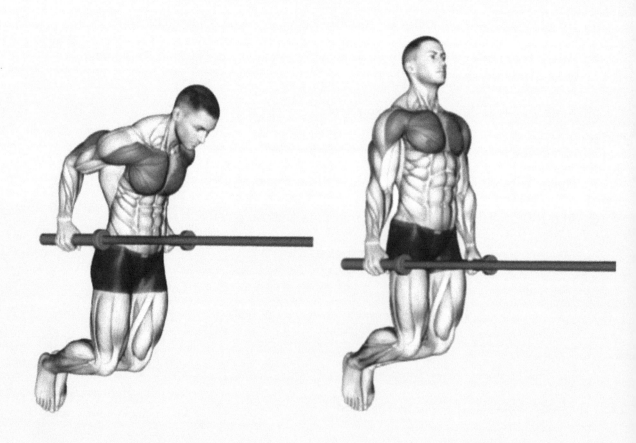

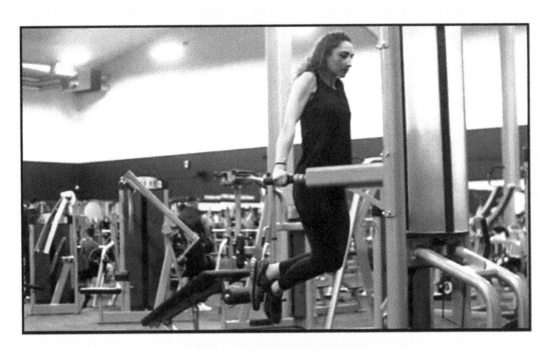

Dips - Starting Position

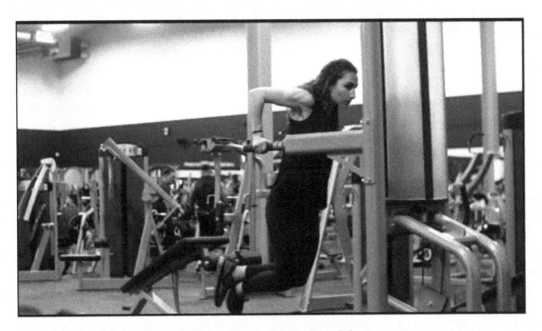

Dips - Finishing Position

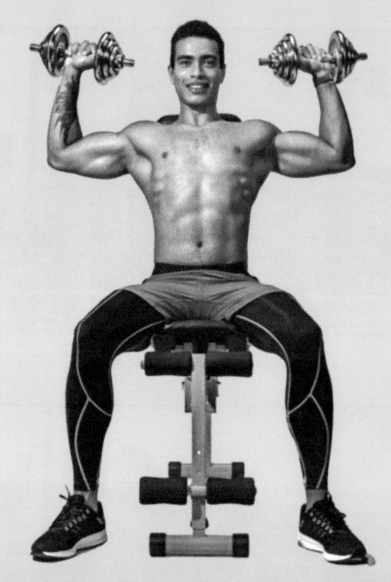

SHOULDER
WORKOUTS

SHOULDER WORKOUTS

MILITARY/OVERHEAD PRESS

ARNOLD DUMBBELL PRESS

SIDE LATERAL RAISES

REAR DELT RAISES

REAR DELT ROWS

DUMBBELL FRONT RAISES

SHOULDER MUSCLES

DELTOIDS
THE DELTOID MUSCLES

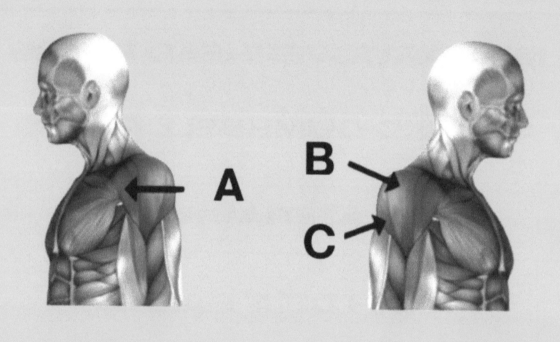

A = ANTERIOR DELTOIDS (FRONT)
B = LATERAL DELTOIDS (SIDE)
C = POSTERIOR DELTOIDS (BACK)

SHOULDER WORKOUTS

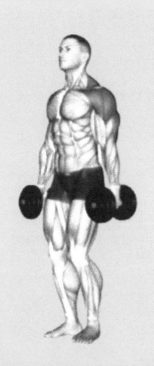 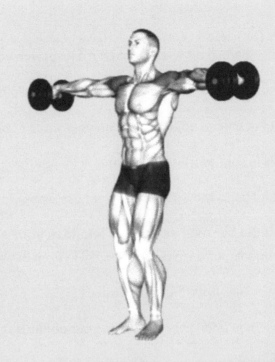

ENTIRE DELTOIDS	ANTERIOR DELTOIDS	LATERAL DELTOIDS	POSTERIOR DELTOIDS
Military/ Overhead Press	Dumbbell Front Raise	Dumbbell Side Lateral Raise	Rear-Delt Raise
Arnold Dumbbell Press			Barbell Rear Delt Row

BARBELL MILITARY/ OVERHEAD PRESS

1. Place barbell on a rack so that it's level with your chest (Figure 11).

2. Grab the bar slightly wider than shoulder width so that the palms are facing up.

3. Lift the barbell up and place on your **upper chest.**

4. This is your **starting position.**

5. Stand back and ensure your **feet are shoulder width apart.**

6. **Lift the bar over your head and lock your arms**. The bar should be level with your anterior deltoids and slightly in front of your head.

7. This is your **finishing position.**

8. Breathe in and lower the bar to your **collar bone.**

9. Lift the bar in a **straight vertical line back up** towards your finishing position as you exhale.

10. As you reach the top of the movement, push your head forwards so that your biceps align closely with your ears (Figure 12).

11. **Lower the bar under control to chin level** and move your head back slightly whilst doing so in order to avoid hitting your forehead on the way down.

12. Repeat.

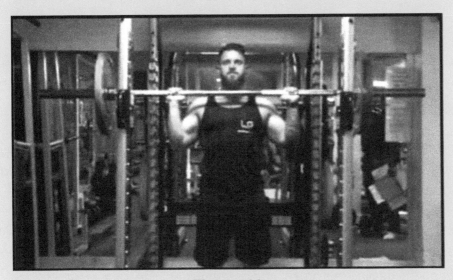

Figure 11:

*Grab the Bar Slightly Wider
than Shoulder Width.*

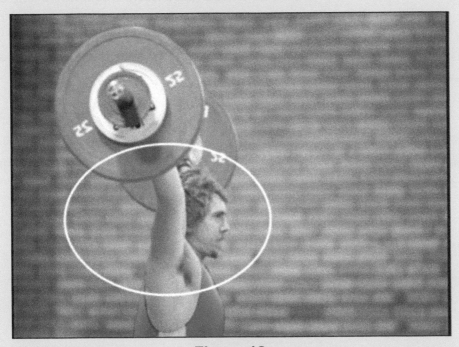

Figure 12:

*Push your head forwards so that
your biceps align closely with your ears*

Military Press vs Overhead Press

- Technically speaking, the main difference between the military press and the overhead press is the position of the feet.

- With the **military press,** the **feet are together**. Think of a soldier standing to attention (military....get it??? lol). The only thing that moves with the military press is your shoulders and arms.

- The **wider base** of the overhead press (where you stand with your feet shoulder width apart) provides a **more stable platform for the lift**. Some people go down too far on the decline movement and risk shoulder injury as a result.

- When you **bring your feet together**, you **reduce** the stability of that **lower-body platform**, which means your **core has to do more work** to keep you stable during the lift, with **your abs and obliques** in particular handling more of the load.

- Therefore, the military press works out your core a lot more than the overhead press.

- The main difference is that the military press is a **strict movement**, testing only upper body strength whilst using your lower body/core strength to support the weight overhead. The overhead press uses a little bit of hip strength to help get the weight overhead.

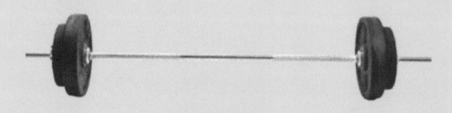

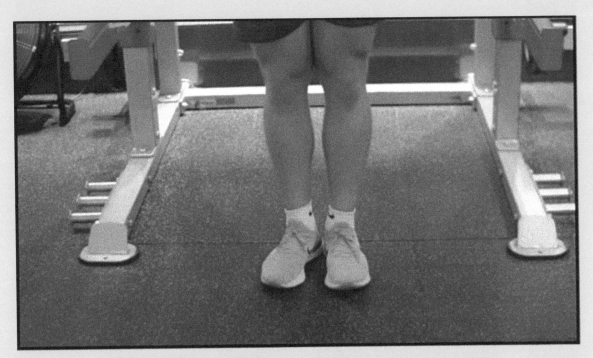

MILITARY PRESS - FEET TOGETHER

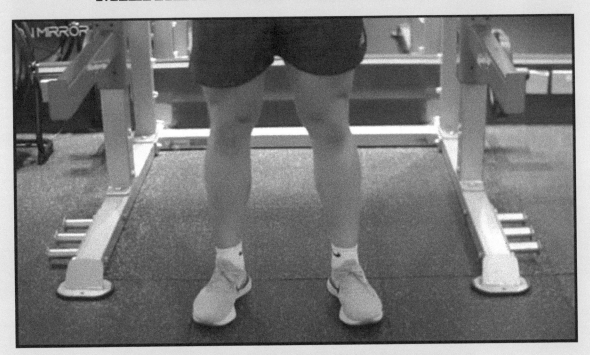

OVERHEAD PRESS - FEET APART

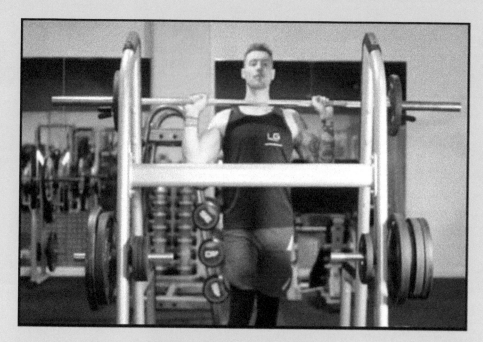

Military/Overhead Press
Starting Position

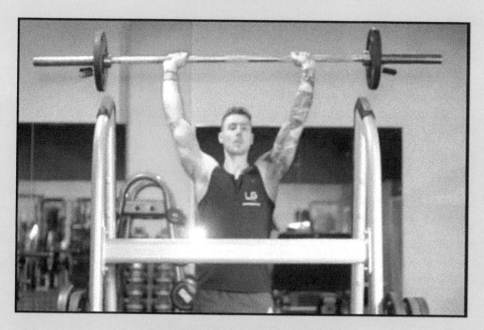

Military/Overhead Press
Finishing Position

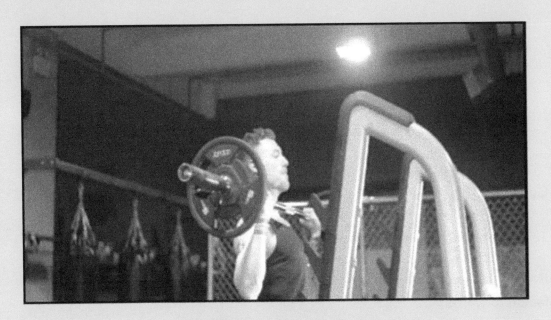

**Military/Overhead Press
Starting Position**

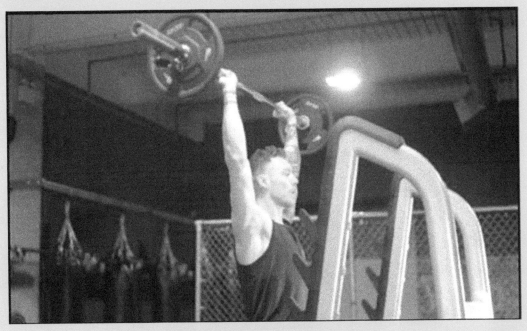

**Military/Overhead Press
Finishing Position**

97

ARNOLD DUMBBELL PRESS

1. Get an exercise bench with back support and sit down.

2. Hold **2 dumbbells with palms facing** you at lower chest level and elbows at level of torso.

3. This is your **starting position.**

4. Raise the **dumbbells and rotate your hands until the palms of your hands are facing forwards.**

5. Continue to lift the dumbbells **until your arms are fully extended and your arm is straight.** Breathe out whilst you're doing this. This is your end position.

6. At the **end position**, the dumbbells are above your shoulders and slightly in front of your head.

7. **Pause at this position for a second** before lowering the dumbbells to its original position by rotating the dumbbells so that the palms are facing you again. Inhale whilst this is being done.

8. Repeat.

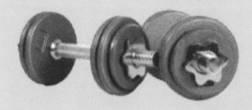

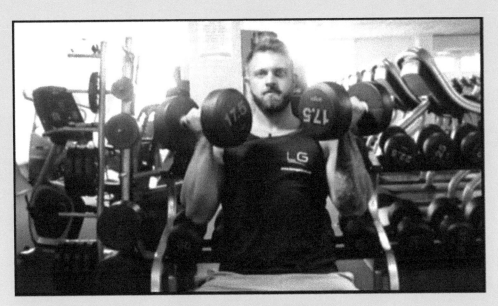

**Arnold Dumbbell Press
Starting Position**

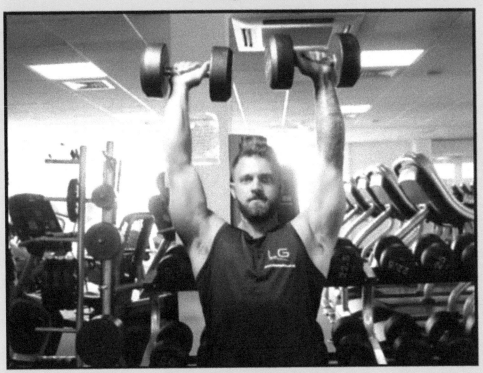

**Arnold Dumbbell Press
Finishing Position**

DUMBBELL SIDE LATERAL RAISES

1. Take one dumbbell in each hand.

2. Stand with a straight torso and dumbbells by your side so that your palms are facing the outer sides of your legs.

3. Keep arms firm but with a slight bend at the elbows.

4. Keep torso firm and body stationary.

5. Lift the dumbbells and hands slightly tilted forwards as if you're pouring water into a cup. Exhale whilst you're doing this.

6. Continue this motion until your arms are parallel to the floor.

7. Hold for a second and then lower the dumbbells as you inhale.

8. Repeat.

Additional Tip: Lateral Delts vs Trapezius Muscles

With this exercise, I would start off with a really light weight in the beginning and lift slowly. As you get above 45 degrees, the trapezius muscles become more active and may start to take over. This defeats the purpose of the exercise (unless you want bigger traps). Instead, try to focus mentally on your shoulder muscles (lateral deltoids) and less on your traps as you raise the weight. If you find this difficult with both weights, then do one hand at a time whilst placing the hand without the weight on the trapezius muscle on the other side to ensure it's soft. Lifting the weight(s) at around 45 degrees in front of your body (ie. **the scapular plane**) also helps activate the lateral deltoids over the trapezius muscles.

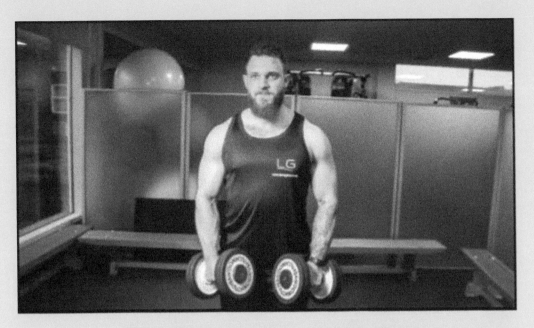

Dumbbell Side Lateral Rise - Starting Position

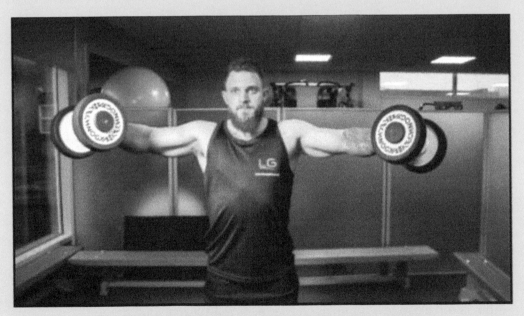

Dumbbell Side Lateral Rise - Finishing Position

101

BARBELL REAR DELT ROW

(PENDLAY ROW VERSION)

The Benefits of The Barbell Row

The Barbell Row exercise helps build your 'traps,' 'upper and middle back,' 'rhomboid,' and 'rear deltoid shoulder' muscles.

How To Perform The Barbell Row

There are **many variations** to this exercise, but the version I suggest starts off with the **barbell on the floor as your starting position** instead of the starting position involving holding the bar from a standing position.

1. Place the barbell onto the floor and stand so that your heels are wider apart than your hips but narrower than shoulders.

2. Ensure you have an overhand grip that's slightly wider than shoulder-width (Figure 13).

3. **Place the barbell over your mid-foot. This is essential for balance** (Figure 14). The most effective way to carry out the barbell row is to lift the weight from the floor to your chest **in a vertical line from this position**. (If the bar starts **over your forefoot** it will pull you forward and out of balance; or it will move back over your mid-foot and hit your knees. If the bar is too close to your shins, however, it will scrape your shins).

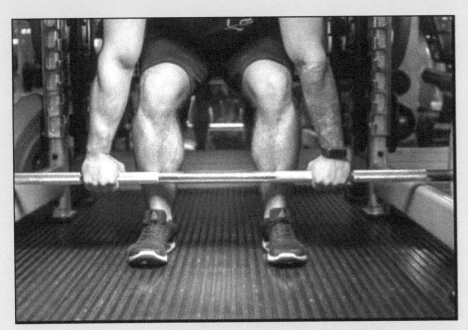

Figure 13:

Overhand Grip for Barbell Row is Wider Than Heels.

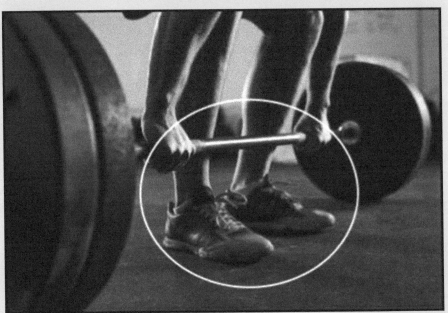

Figure 14:

Place the barbell over your mid-foot. This is essential for balance.

4. Keep your **core tight and feet flat on the floor**. Point your knees outward away from bar so that you **don't hit your knees during the lift**. A 30 degree angle is sufficient.

5. With only a **slight bend in your knees**, push your hips backward (as if you were trying to close a car door) until your hands grab the bar.

> **NOTE**: Your legs should be slightly bent with the knees unlocked. You should feel a stretch in your hamstrings.

6. Elevate your chest to a 45 degree angle.

7. Bend over whilst keeping a natural arch on your back.

8. Straighten your arms downwards so you're preparing for an upwards lift. As you do so, **imagine there's a lemon underneath your armpits that you're trying to squeeze**. This will activate your lats and prevent your back from rounding.

9. Lift up in a vertical line whilst 'squeezing the lemon,' keeping your elbows close to your hips and moving upwards until the bar touches your chest.

10. Return the bar **quickly to the floor after it hits your chest**. It's almost as if you're dropping the bar to the floor (but you're not!!!). **It must go down faster than it went up**. Don't lower it slowly to feel your muscles more. **You're working them during the upward movement which matters most on Barbell Rows** (like on Deadlifts (see later).

Again let me reiterate, this doesn't mean you should drop the bar.
You should hold it as you go down, **but lower it fast.**

11.   Bring the bar back to your starting position and repeat.

<u>Additional Tips</u>

- **Don't look up** when doing this exercise. This squeezes the spinal discs in your neck and can injure it. **Don't look down at your feet** either or your back will round. **Keep your head inline with the rest of your spine**. From the side you should have a straight line from your head to your hips.

- **Pull the weight from the floor against your lower chest**, then return it to the floor for each rep. Don't hold the bar in the air between reps.

- **To prevent your lower back from rounding**, lift your chest towards the ceiling at a 45 degree angle whilst setting up and squeeze your lats (remember the lemon under the armpits) to lock your chest in position.

- A common variation of this exercise involves **NOT** resetting between reps and only lowering the bar a few inches above the floor (like a Romanian deadlift). **This is also fine, but it's probably safer to use lighter weights for this variation.**

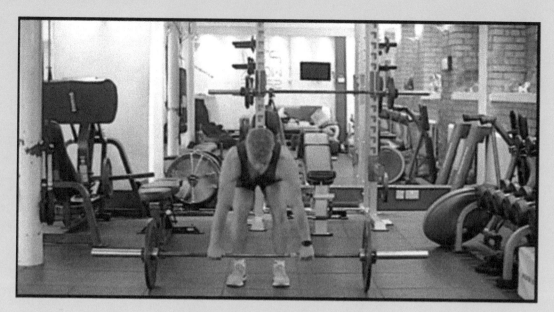

Pendlay Row - Starting Position

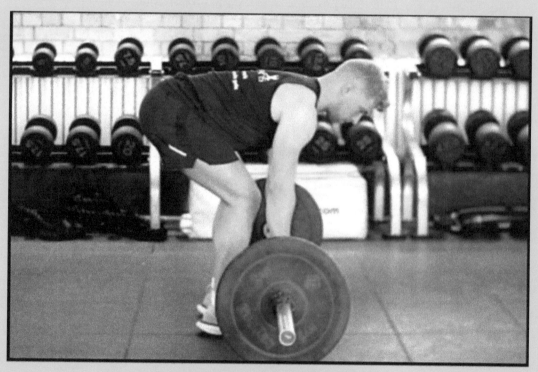

Pendlay Row - Starting Position

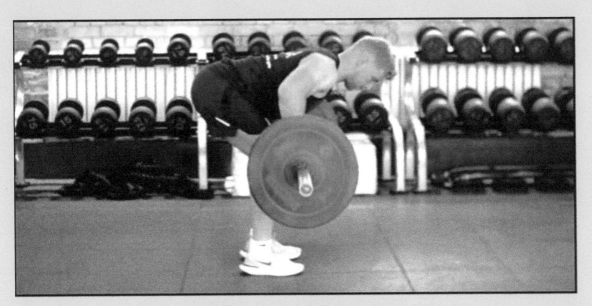

Pendlay Row - Mid-Position

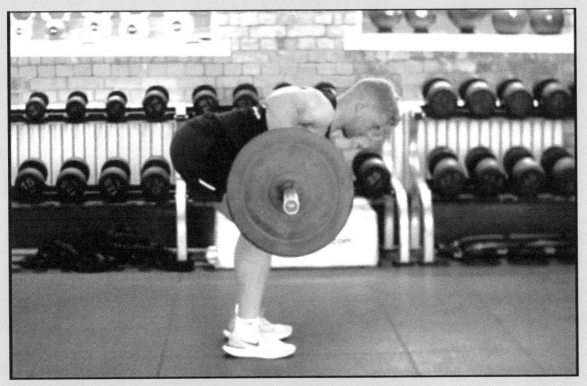

Pendlay Row - Finishing Position

107

DUMBBELL FRONT RAISE

1. Pick up a couple of dumbbells and stand upright.

2. **Keep torso tight and firm**. Dumbbells should be level with thighs so that the palms of your hands are facing your body.

3. Lift the right dumbbell, whilst **ensuring the body is firm** (i.e., no swinging).

4. Continue this movement in an arc of motion going upwards and forwards away from your body **until your arms are parallel to the floor.**

5. **Palms should be facing down at all times**. Ensure you're exhaling during this time.

6. Pause for a second at this position and then slowly bring back to starting position.

7. Do the same with the left arm as you're bringing right arm back to starting position.

8. Repeat.

Additional Tips

- You can also lift the dumbbells at the same time if you feel more comfortable doing so.

- Alternatively, this exercise can also be done using a barbell.

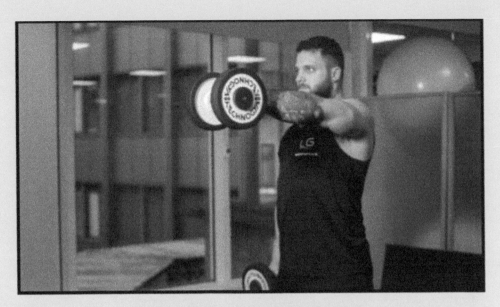

Alternate Dumbbell Front Raise
(Left Hand)

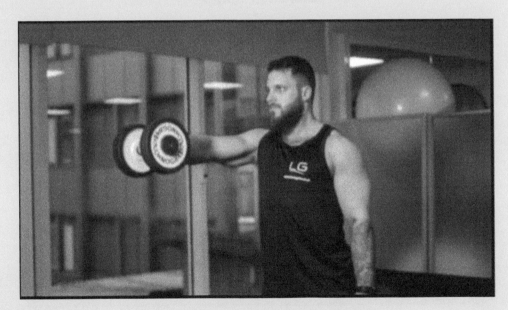

Alternate Dumbbell Front Raise
(Right Hand)

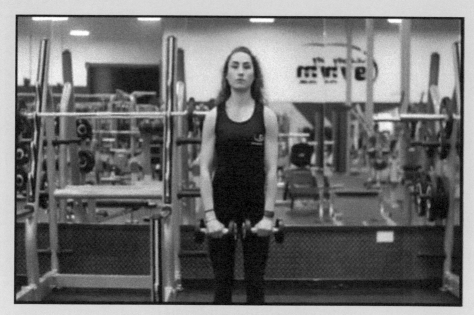

Dumbbell Front Raise

Starting Position

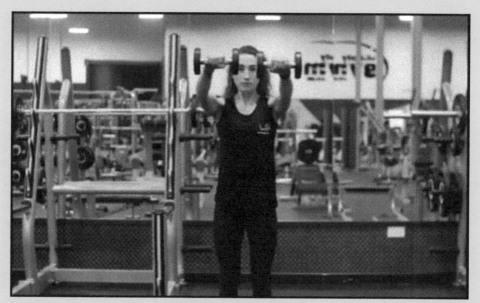

Dumbbell Front Raise

Finishing Position

110

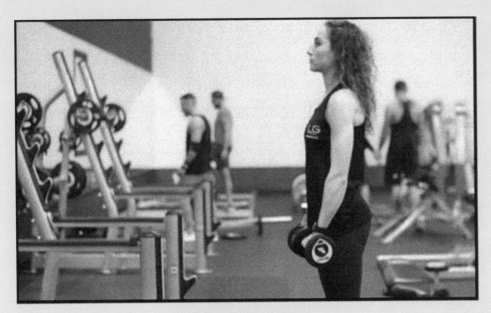

Dumbbell Front Raise
Starting Position

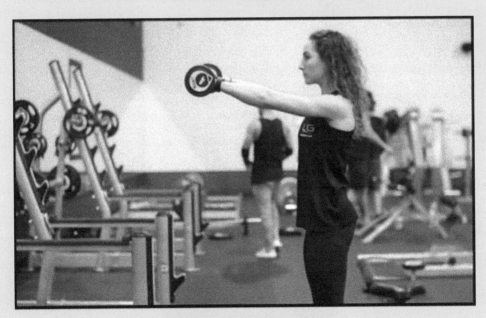

Dumbbell Front Raise
Finishing Position

111

SEATED REAR DELT RAISE

This is a great exercise for the **back of the shoulders (rear deltoids)**.

1. Sit at the end of the bench.

2. **Bend at the waist** but keep back straight and firm.

3. Pick up the dumbbells with **each hand so the palms are facing each other**.

4. Keep torso firm and arms slightly bent at the elbows.

5. Make sure your legs are together and the dumbbells are behind your calves. This will be your starting position.

6. Exhale as you lift the dumbbells to the side.

7. Continue until **both arms are parallel to the floor**. Ensure that only your arms are moving. The rest of the **body should be still.**

8. **Pause at the top of the movement** before lowering the dumbbells back to start position.

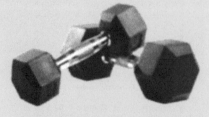

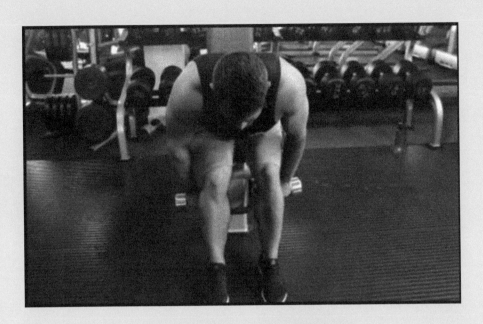

Seated Rear Delt Raise
Starting Position

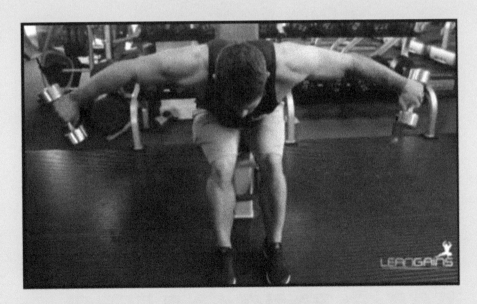

Seated Rear Delt Raise
Finishing Position

113

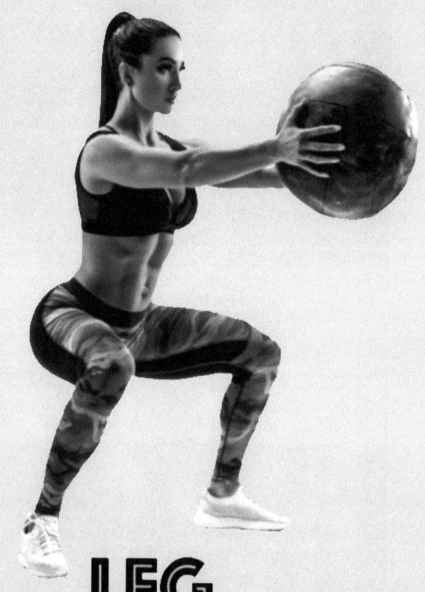

LEG
WORKOUTS

LEG WORKOUTS

BARBELL SQUATS

BARBELL FRONT SQUATS

LEG PRESS

DUMBBELL LUNGE

BARBELL LUNGE

ROMANIAN DEADLIFT

UPPER LEG MUSCLES

(QUADS AND HAMSTRINGS)

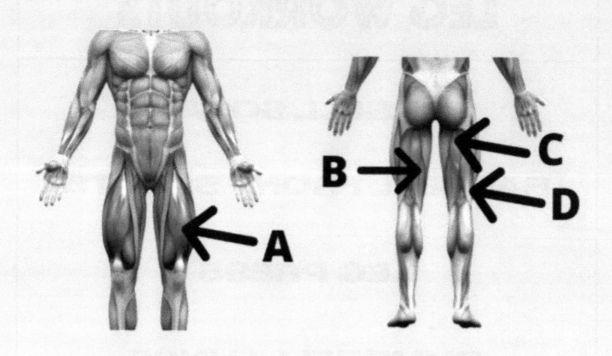

A = QUADRICEPS (QUADS) (Thigh Muscles)

B = SEMIMEMBRANOSUS   (Hamstring)

C = SEMITENDINOSUS   (Hamstring)

D = BICEP FEMORIS   (Hamstring)

LEG WORKOUTS

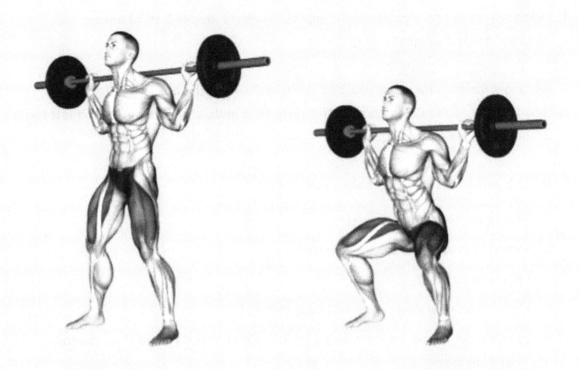

QUADS & HAMSTRINGS	QUADS	HAMSTRINGS
Barbell Squats	Barbell Front Squats	Romanian Deadlifts
Barbell Lunges		
Dumbbell Lunges		
Leg Press		

BARBELL SQUATS

1. Place the barbell on a power/squat rack so level with **upper half of chest**, and load the desired weight.

2. Go under the bar and place your heels/feet shoulder-width apart and slightly position feet at an outward angle. **The right foot should be 1 o'clock and left foot should be 11 o'clock** (Figure 15).

3. Ensure you do the following before you un-rack:

   • Grip the bar with a narrow grip,

   • Bring your shoulder blades together,

   • Raise your chest,

   • Straighten your lower back and keep firm,

   • Put the bar below the bone at the top of your shoulder blades (i.e., **on top of your traps**).

4. Un-rack the bar by straightening legs and taking 2 steps back, and maintain the above squatting posture (raised chest, narrow grip, etc.)

5. Pick a spot on the floor 6-feet in front of you and **keep staring at that imaginary spot** during the entire set. This will help maintain your posture and reduce risk of

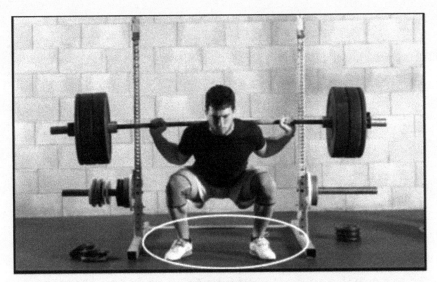

Figure 15:

*Slightly slightly position feet at an outward angle.
The right foot should be 1 o'clock and left foot
should be 11 o'clock.*

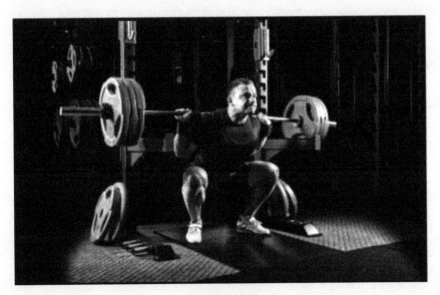

Figure 16:

*At the Bottom of the Squat, you want your Hips to be
back and Slightly Lower than your Knee Caps.*

6. Take a deep breath and commence your downward motion whilst:

   - Hips are back,

   - Chest is up,

   - Back is straight and tight.

7. As you squat down, stick your hips and butt outwards as if you're about to sit on a chair.

8. Squat down until your hip is below your waist (i.e., beyond the point at which your thighs are parallel to the floor). In other words, **at the bottom of the squat, you want your hips to be back and slightly lower than your knee caps** (Figure 16). This allows for a fuller range of motion and will **incorporate more of your gluteal muscles** as well.

9. From this bottom position, drive your butt straight upwards without moving forward, and drive your heels into the floor to allow you to lift back up to starter position until legs are straight.

10. Repeat.

Additional Tips

- Make sure your feet are flat on the floor at all times.

- Drive though the heels. Keep pressure through the heels at all times.

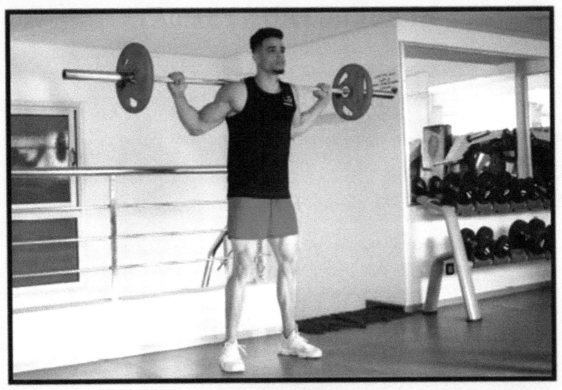

Barbell Squat
Starting Position

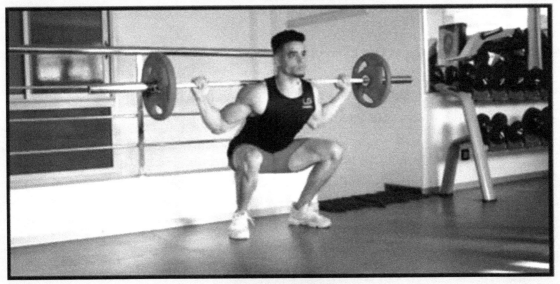

Barbell Squat
Finishing Position

BARBELL FRONT SQUATS

1. Similar to the back squat, the stance should be very similar [i.e., Feet should be shoulder width apart and at an angle (11 o'clock and 1 o'clock)].

2. However, instead of placing the bar on the traps, you're placing the bar on your front shoulders.

3. There are 2 options when it comes to gripping the bar (**Figure 17 and 18**):

    1) The **'Clean Grip'**: Hold barbell against the front of your shoulders with both palms facing upwards. This creates a lot of stress on the wrists for some people (this is especially the case for those with poor wrist flexibility). So if this is the case with you, then try removing thumb and little finger from the bar and grip with the remaining fingers. Alternatively, use the 'bodybuilder' grip [see below]

    2) The **'Bodybuilder Grip'**: Hold the barbell on your front shoulders, cross your arms over and grab the bar so palms are facing downwards. Then lift your elbows.

4. Keep your back straight and torso upright.

5. Take a deep breath, keep your core firm, push your hips back and squat keeping your knees in line with your toes.

6. Continue until thighs are just below parallel to the ground. As you're going down, remember to keep your feet flat on the ground.

7. When it comes to the lift, use the heels and butt to drive the bar back to the starting position. Keep your chest and elbows up whilst doing this.

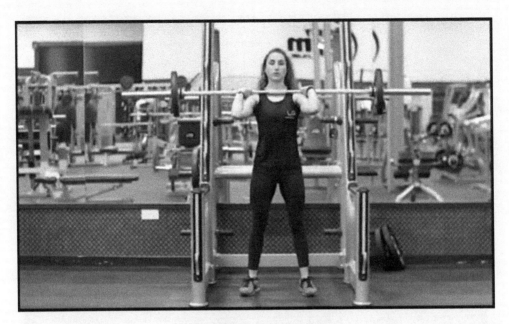

Barbell Front Squat
Starting Position

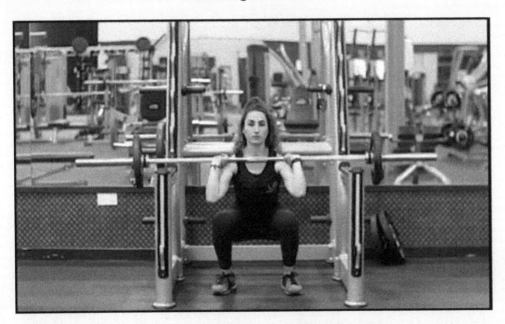

Barbell Front Squat
Finishing Position

123

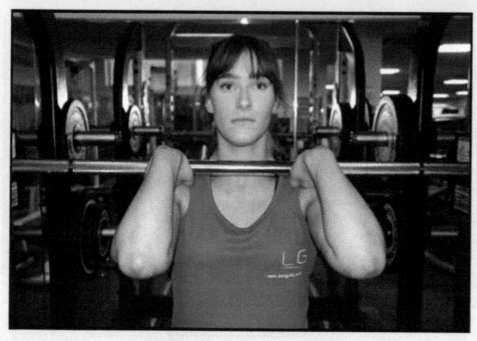

Figure 17: The 'Clean' Grip

Hold barbell against the front of your shoulders with both palms facing upwards.

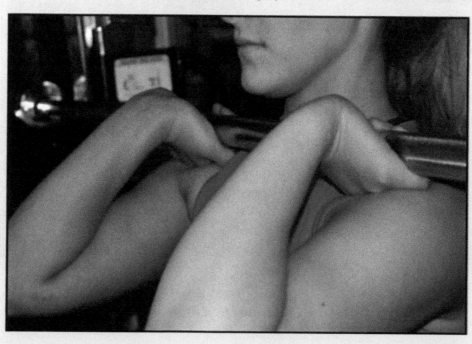

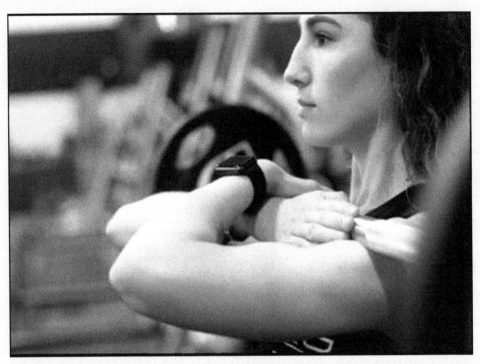

Figure 18: The 'Bodybuilder' Grip

Hold the barbell on your front shoulders, cross your arms over and grab the bar so palms are facing downwards. Then lift your elbows.

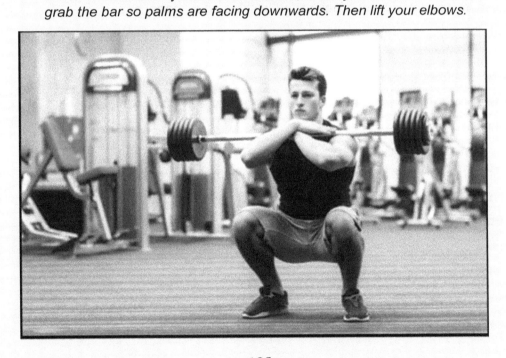

LEG PRESS

1. Select the desired weight.

2. Place your feet slightly wider than hip width apart ((Figure 19a). Your legs should be at least but ideally 90 degree angle to your knees. Your knees should be in line with your feet and neither be bowed inward nor outward

3. **Ensure your lower back and butt** remain in contact with the seat at all times during the movements.

4. Grab handles on either side of the machine for safely if you're new to this exercise.

5. Push the weight with your feet without locking your knees, and turn the locking safety handle allowing the machine to move.

6. Push the weight with your feet, but ensure you never lock your knees out fully (as this would create a lot of stress on the knee joints).

7. Bring your **knees back towards your chest**, make sure your **feet remain flat against the plate** at all times whilst doing so (Figure 19b).

8. Repeat.

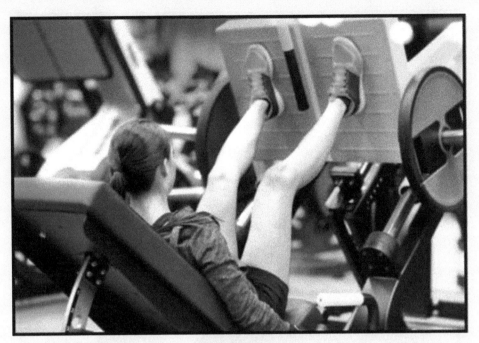

Leg Press
Starting Position

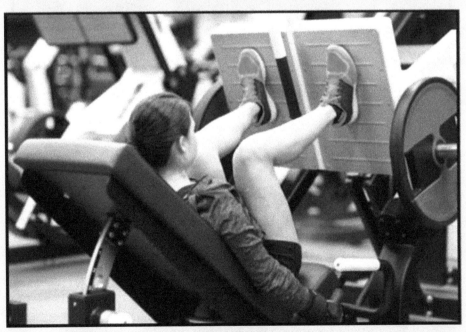

Leg Press
Finishing Position

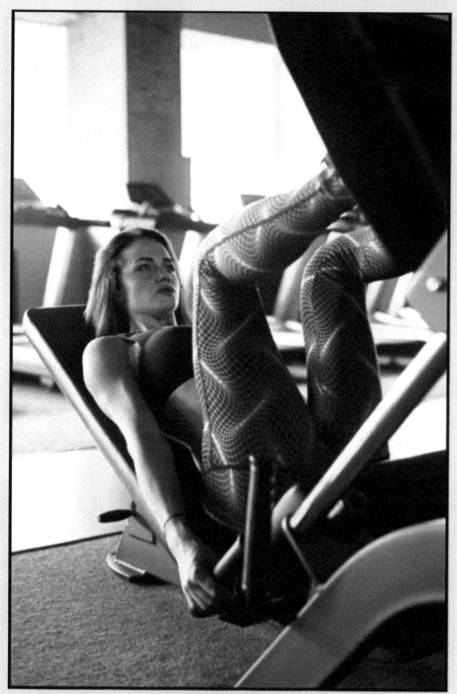

Figure 19a:

*Ensure your feet are slightly wider than hip width apart.
Your knees should be in line with your feet and neither
be bowed inward nor outward.*

Additional Tips

- Ensure your knees **don't** lock at the end of the rep. Instead, keep your legs slightly bent at the knee on extension.

- Do not bow your knees inwards or outwards.

- Keep them aligned with your feet. Push from your heals and not the toes.

- Placing your hands behind your head during the movement allows for a deeper contraction of the muscles once you've got used to this exercise.

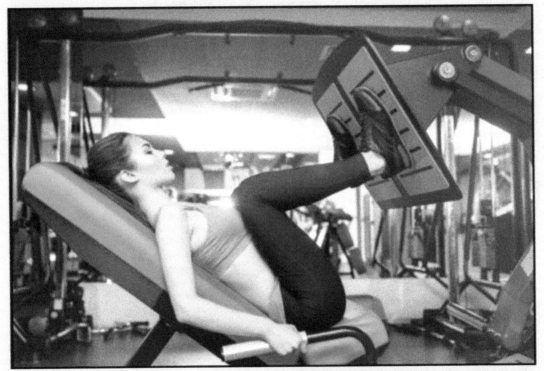

Figure 19b:

Bring your Knees Back towards your Chest, and Make Sure Your Feet Remain Flat against the Plate at All Times whilst doing so.

DUMBBELL LUNGE

1. Stand upright holding a pair of dumbbells with a slight bend in the knees.

2. Ensure dumbbells are at the side of your body with **palms facing outer thighs**.

3. Step forward with your right leg until your **thigh is parallel to the floor**.

4. Your left leg (your back leg) should be bent in a way whereby the **knee is almost touching the floor.**

5. Keep your torso straight and upright with your head up. Don't allow your right knee to overshoot your toes.

6. Push yourself back to the starting position using your heel to **drive you**.

7. Repeat using the left leg.

Additional Tips

- Ensure your knees don't exceed your toes (Figure 20).
- Do not bow your knees inwards or outwards.
- Keep your back straight, firm, and head up at all times.

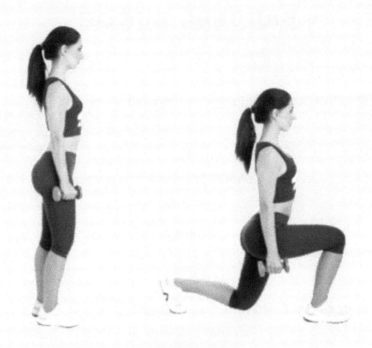

Figure 20:

*Ensure Your Knees **Don't** Exceed your Toes.*

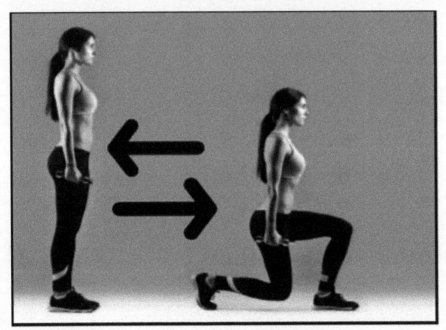

Dumbbell Lunge Exercise

131

BARBELL LUNGE

1. This is **similar to the dumbbell lunge**, but instead, we're using a barbell.

2. Position the barbell just **below shoulder level** within a squat rack.

3. Just like the barbell squat, position the barbell on your traps and take a few steps back.

4. Ensure your **torso is tight and firm**, take a deep breath and lunge your **right foot forwards** until **parallel to the floor** ensuring your hip is taking the main brunt of the weight.

5. The left leg (back leg) should bend in such a way that the left knee is almost touching the floor.

6. Make sure you're in an upright position and that your **knee does not go in front of your toes (Figure 21).**

7. Exhale as you lift up making sure that the weight is transferred to your heels as you're coming back up to the starting position.

8. Repeat using the **left leg**.

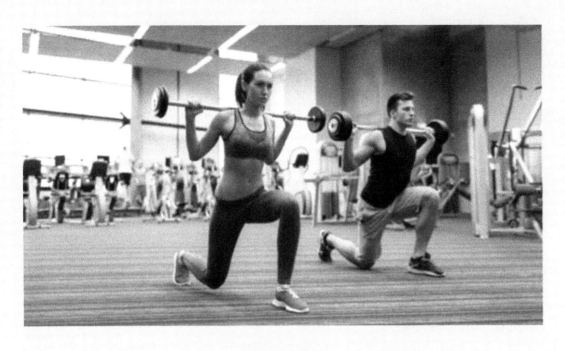

Figure 21:

Make Sure Knees Don't Go in Front of Toes.
Don't Bow Knees Inwards or Outwards.

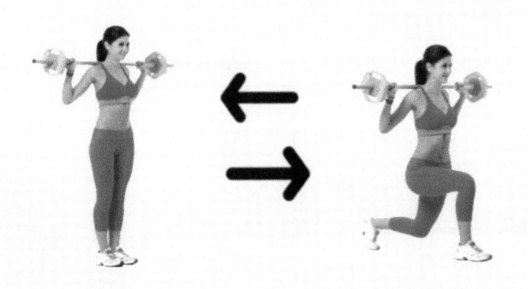

__ROMANIAN DEADLIFT__

The Romanian deadlift is similar to the conventional barbell deadlift but it targets your **hamstrings and glutes** more than the back.

There are 3 Stages involved in the Romanian Deadlift.

They consist of:

A) The Set-Up.

B) Raising The Bar.

C) The Descent.

A. __The Set Up__

1. Place barbell on the **floor**.

2. Stand upright with feet **hip-width apart**. Stand **as close as you can** in front of the barbell so your **shins are almost touching the bar**. (If you are too far away from the bar, you will end up leaning forward to reach it. This can throw your back out of alignment).

3. Ensure the bar is over your **mid-foot** region.

4. **Bend** your knees slightly.

5. Grab the barbell with an overhand grip (palms facing down) with arms roughly shoulder-width apart so that they're slightly outside the legs **(Figure 22).**

6. **Ensure your back and core are tight. Flex the muscles in your shoulders, upper back, and abs** while you lift the barbell. This allows you to keep good form as you lift and lower the weight. At the same time, **press your upper arms into your sides (lats) as if you were trying to crush a couple of lemons in your armpits.**

B. Raising The Bar

7. Maintain a firm posture and **keep your back straight with chest upwards** at roughly a 45 degree angle **(Figure 23)**.

8. Begin breathing out as you start moving the bar upwards, and **maintain close contact with your body** at all times. Do not rush this movement.

9. During the ascent, **contract your glutes** to help push your hips towards the bar.

10. Straighten your body by **standing up gradually** as the bar travels back up your legs.

11. Stand up tall with your **back and neck straight yet still firm.**

C. The Descent

12. This is your **starting position** for consequent reps (Figure 24).

13. During this movement, make sure the bar is still as close as possible to your thighs. Keep your core and muscles tight (remember to squeeze those lemons underneath your armpits).

14. **Fix your gaze** on a spot about 10 feet away. Take a deep breath and keep focussed on the spot (i.e., **don't look down**).

15. Bend at the waist and **slowly** lower the bar by shifting your **hips and butt backwards** away from the bar. As you do, bend over the bar.

16. **Keep the bar close to your legs as if you're rolling the bar down them towards your ankles**. Stop the descent when you can't go any further without bending your knees more. (For most people, this is when the bar is below the knees, and they **often start to feel a stretch along the backs of their legs** by this point).

17. Keep your arms still and shoulders back during the descent.

18. Repeat.

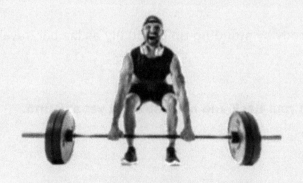

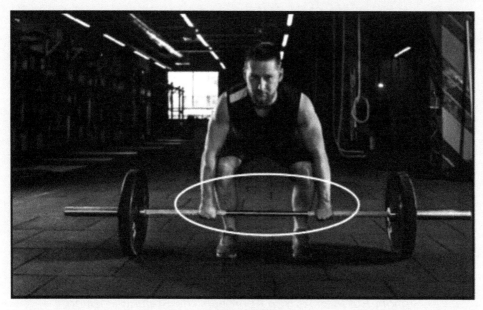

Figure 22:
*Grab the barbell with an overhand grip with arms
roughly shoulder-width so they're slightly outside the legs*

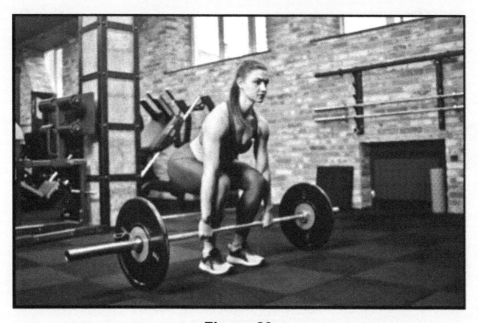

Figure 23:
*Maintain a firm posture and keep your back straight with
chest upwards at roughly a 45-degree angle.*

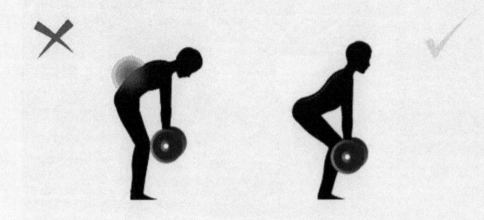

Figure 24:

*Keep Your Core Tight, Chest Up, Back and Neck
Straight But Firm As You Approach The Starting Position.*

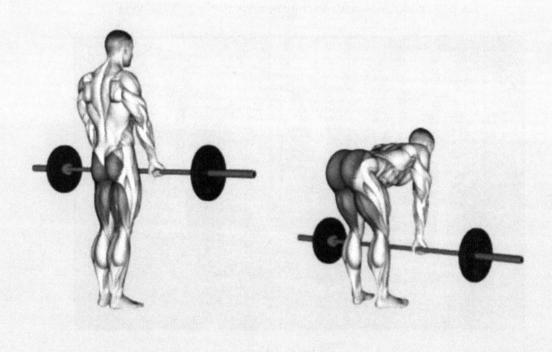

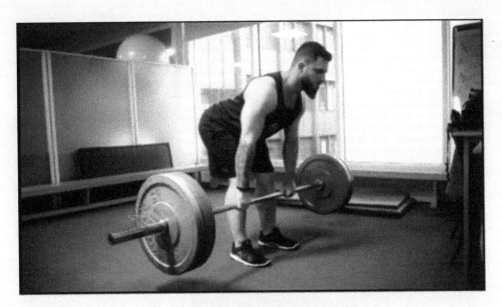

Romanian Deadlift
Starting Position

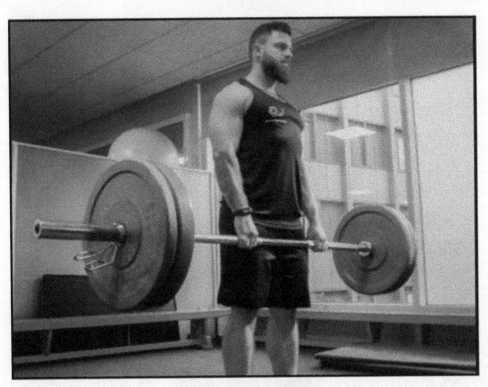

Romanian Deadlift
Finishing Position

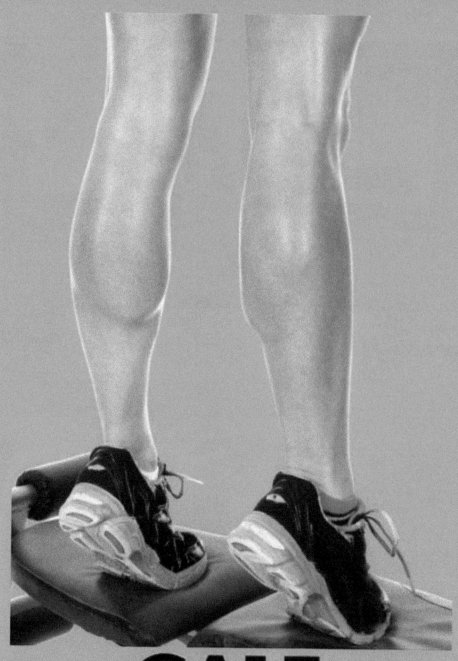

CALF
WORKOUTS

CALF WORKOUTS

STANDING CALF RAISES

SEATED CALF RAISES

CALF RAISES ON LEG PRESS

CALF MUSCLES

(LOWER LEG MUSCLES)

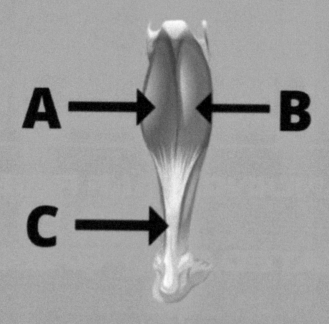

A = GASTROCNEMIUS (MEDIAL)   (Inner Calf)

B = GASTROCNEMIUS (LAT)   (Outer Calf)

C = ACHILLES TENDON   (Not a Muscle)

CALF WORKOUTS

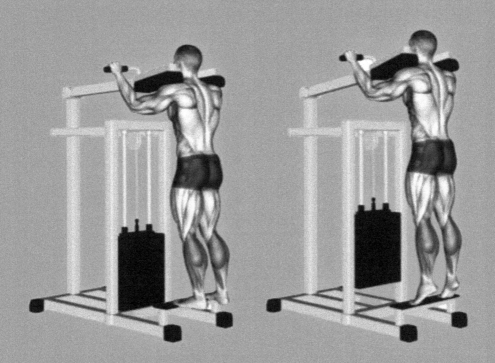

CALF MUSCLES
Standing Calf Raises
Seated Calf Raises
Calf Raises on Leg Press

STANDING CALF RAISES

1. **Pick barbell up from squat rack** (as if you're about to do a squat) and **place on your traps**.

2. Use a **sturdy elevated surface** so that your **heels are elevated off the ground** (Figure 25). Most people do this by placing a 'step platform' or, if one's not available, a large weight on the floor.

3. **Keep torso tight**, stand with the balls of your feet on the elevated surface and push up as high as you can until your heels are in the air.

4. Return back to the **starting position** slowly.

5. Repeat.

Additional Tips

1. If you're new to this, it's much safer to perform this exercise using a **smith machine** (Figure 27).

2. Alternatively, some gyms have a **'standing calf raise machine'** (Figure 26) which is also an excellent alternative.

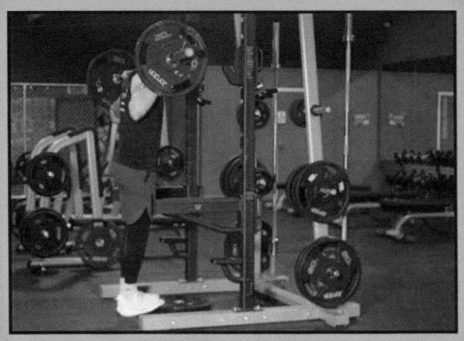

<u>Barbell Calf Raise</u>
Starting Position

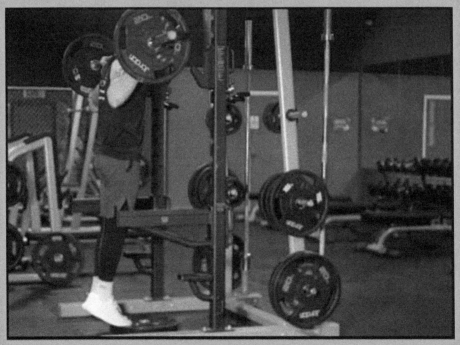

<u>Barbell Calf Raise</u>
Finishing Position

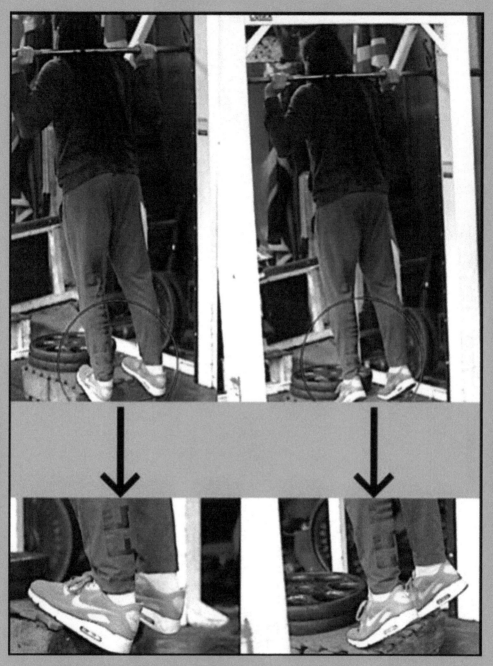

Figure 25:

Use a sturdy elevated surface so that your heels are elevated off the ground.

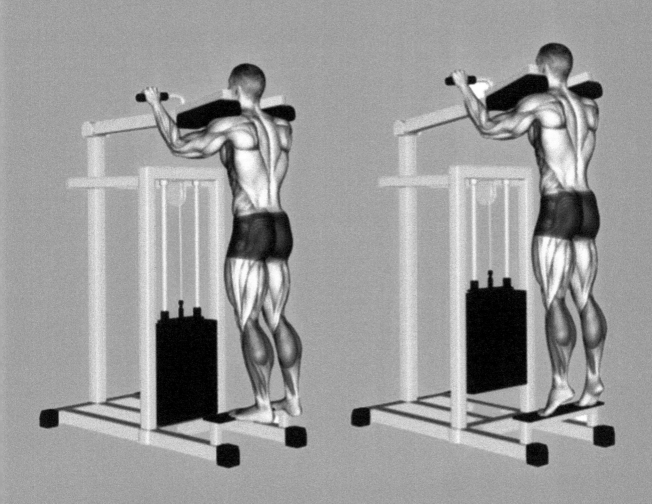

Figure 26:

*A 'Standing Calf-Raise' Machine is an excellent
alternative to the weighted-barbell.*

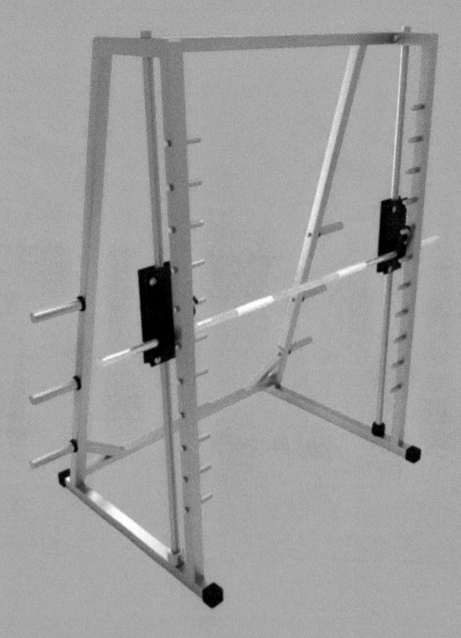

Figure 27:

*Using a Smith Machine for this
exercise is a much safer option.*

SEATED CALF RAISES

1. Select desired weight.

2. Sit down in machine and **place balls of feet**/toes on the platform so **heels are hanging behind**.

3. Adjust lever pad to accommodate the thickness of your legs and **place over thighs**.

4. Inhale whilst **gradually lowering your heels and bending at the ankles**. You should stop when you feel your calves are fully stretched.

5. Exhale whilst returning towards the starting position. Stop this upwards movement when calves are fully contracted.

6. Hold at the **top position** for about a second and then repeat.

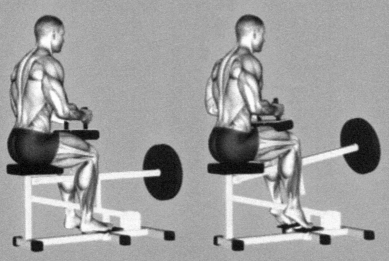

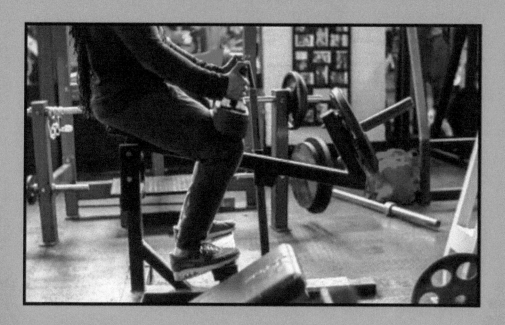

<u>Seated Calf Raise</u>
Starting Position

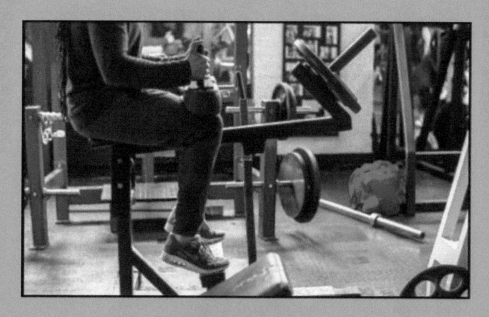

<u>Seated Calf Raise</u>
Starting Position

CALF RAISES ON LEG PRESS

- Similar to conventional leg press, the main difference here is that we're using the same machine to train our calves.

1. Select weight, sit down in machine and **place your feet on the plate**. Ensure your butt is tucked snugly against the back rest.

2. Lower the safety bars, press the plate all the way up and then extend your legs, but **do not lock your knees**.

3. Ensure a 90 degree angle between your torso and your legs.

4. Move your feet down the plate so that the only part of your feet touching the plate are your toes/balls of your feet. Your heels should be hanging off the plate.

5. Inhale as you allow your heels to come down slightly **until you feel a stretch in your calves**. This will be your **starting position**.

6. From here, **raise your heels by pressing on the platform**, exhale and flex your calves **keeping your knee stationary at all times**.

7. Repeat.

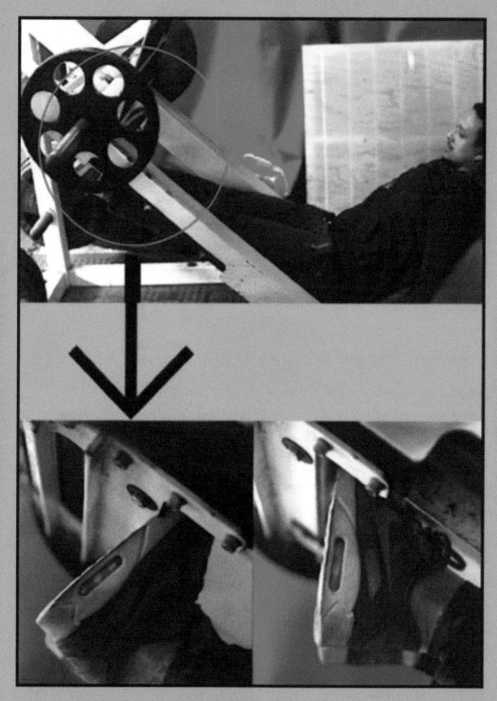

**Calf-Raise on
Leg-Press Machine**

Additional Tips

- You can move your toes to an outward position (10 o'clock on the left and 2 o'clock on the right) to workout the inner portion of your calves.

- Turn your calves slightly inwards to focus on the outer portion of your calves.

- A more challenging version of this exercise is to work on one leg/calf at a time

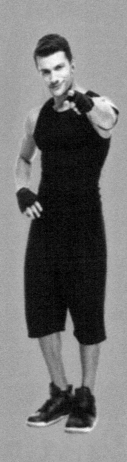

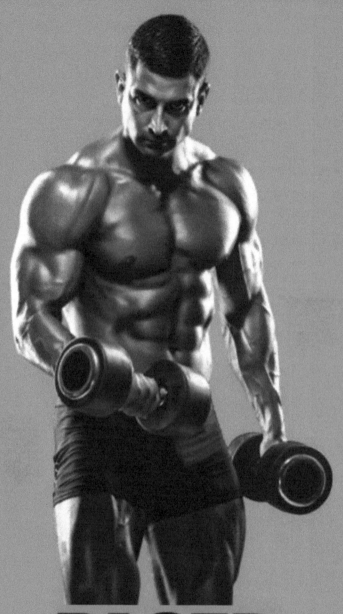

BICEP WORKOUTS

BICEP WORKOUTS

BARBELL BICEP CURL

E-Z BARBELL BICEP CURL

HAMMER CURL

DUMBBELL CURL

CHIN-UPS

BICEP MUSCLES

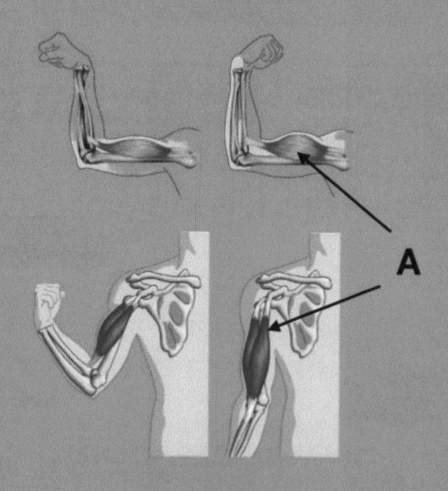

A = BICEPS BRACHII

The biceps muscle has two heads,
the short head and the long head.

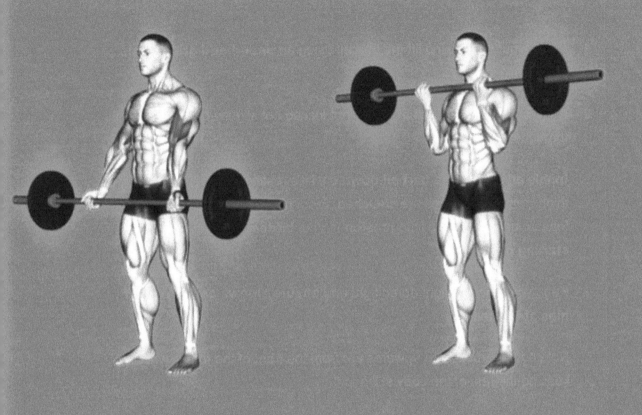

BICEP WORKOUTS
Barbell Bicep Curl
E-Z Barbell Bicep Curl
Hammer Curl
Dumbbell Curl
Chin-Ups

BARBELL BICEP CURLS

1. Select your weight and lift the barbell using an **underhand grip (palms facing upwards).**

2. Make sure your legs and arms are not locked but slightly bent at the joints throughout.

3. **Inhale and lower the barbell down** until it's resting on the front of your thighs, and your biceps are stretched. From here, bring the bar slightly forward until you feel a little **tension** in your biceps. This will be your **starting position**.

4. Keep your back straight, torso tight and **ensure elbows are in front of hips at all times**.

5. Rotate the barbell in an upwards arc from the front of the thighs whilst keeping the rest of the body still and firm.

6. Stop when you have reached the **chest area** and contracted your biceps (Figure 28). Hold for a second or so in this position before bringing the barbell back down.

7. **Never let the barbell touch your thighs or chest** during the actual movement in order to keep the tension within the bicep muscle.

8. Repeat.

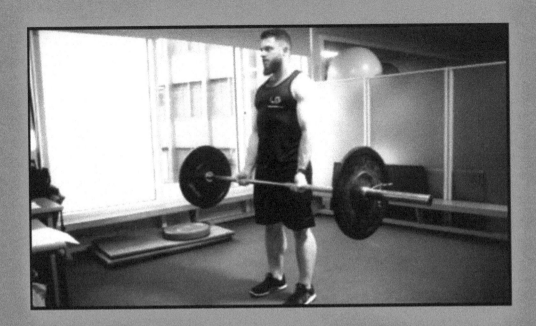

Barbell Biceps Curl
Starting Position

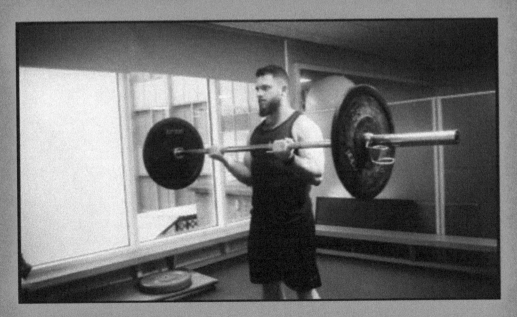

Barbell Biceps Curl
Finishing Position

159

E-Z BARBELL BICEP CURLS

- The E-Z barbell curl is **virtually identical** to the straight barbell curl, but the main difference is the **angulation of your hands which are more pronated**. In other words, the thumbs are higher than the little finger. This takes the pressure off your wrists and elbows.

- The E-Z bar is more ideal, therefore, for those who have had or are more prone to wrist/elbow injuries. The traditional straight barbell curl is thought to be more effective overall for training biceps, but they're both great exercise routines.

1. Select your weight and lift the E-Z barbell **using an underhand grip (palms facing upwards).**

2. Make sure your legs and arms are **not locked** but slightly bent at the joints throughout.

3. Inhale and lower the barbell down until it's resting on the front of your thighs, and your **biceps are stretched**. From here, bring the bar slightly forward until you feel a little tension in your biceps. This will be your starting position.

4. Keep your back straight, torso tight and ensure elbows are in front of hips at all times.

5. Rotate the barbell in an upwards arc from the front of the thighs whilst keeping the rest of the body still and firm.

6. Stop when you have reached the **chest area** and contracted your biceps. Hold for a second or so in this position before bringing the barbell back down.

7. Never let the barbell touch your thighs or chest during the actual movement in order to keep the tension within the bicep muscle.

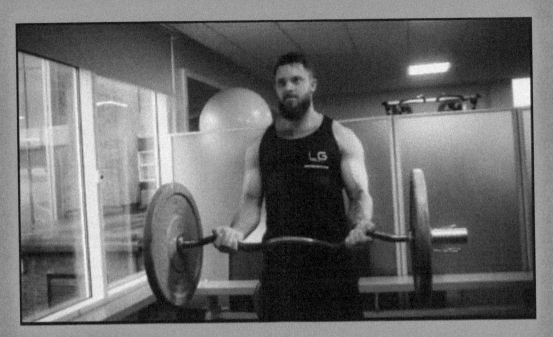

E-Z Bicep Curl
Starting Position

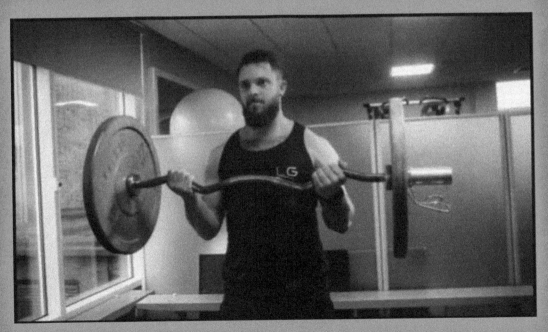

E-Z Bicep Curl
Finishing Position

161

BICEP DUMBBELL CURLS

1. Stand up straight with **feet shoulder width apart** and with a dumbbell on each side at arms length.

2. The palms of your hands should be **facing away from you**.

3. Hold **dumbbells in the middle** and ensure there's a slight bend in your elbows.

4. Keep your **elbows in front of your hips** throughout the exercise.

5. Keep upper arms firm, exhale and curl weight along a forward arc towards the chest so as to **contract the bicep**s.

6. Ensure biceps are fully contracted whilst raising the dumbbells until they're just passed 90 degrees at **around shoulder level**.

7. Squeeze and hold for a second.

8. Inhale and return slowly back to starting position making sure you're maintaining tension within.

9. Repeat.

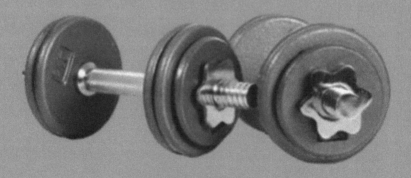

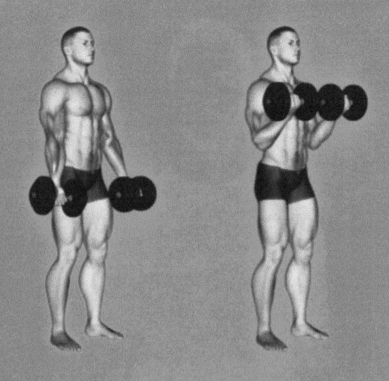

Bicep Dumbbell Curl

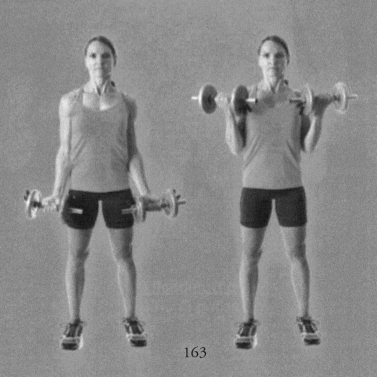

163

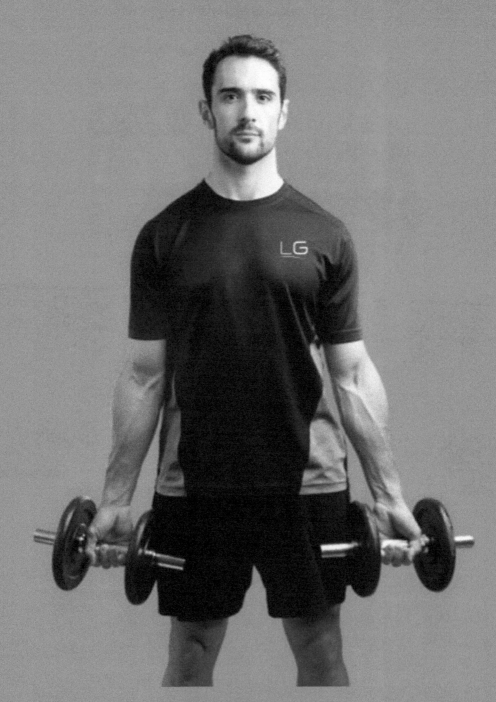

Bicep Dumbbell Curl
Starting Position

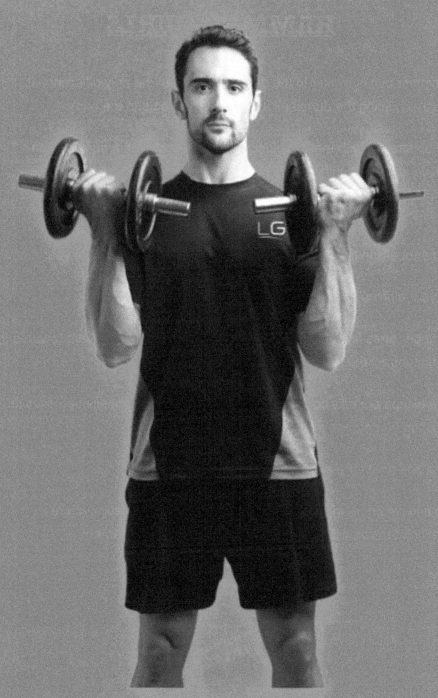

Bicep Dumbbell Curl
Finishing Position

__HAMMER CURLS__

- The hammer curl is similar to the dumbbell curl, but the only difference is that you're holding the dumbbell at a 90 degree angle to the body.

1. Stand up straight with feet shoulder width apart and with a dumbbell on each side at arms length.

2. The palms of your hands should be facing your torso.

3. Hold dumbbells in the middle and ensure there's a slight bend in your elbows.

4. Keep your elbows in front of your hips throughout the exercise.

5. Keep upper arms firm, exhale and curl weight along a forward arc towards the chest so as to contract the biceps.

6. Ensure biceps are fully contracted whilst raising the dumbbells until they're just passed 90 degrees at around shoulder level.

7. Squeeze and hold for a second.

8. Inhale and return slowly back to starting position making sure you're maintaining tension within the biceps throughout the movement.

9. Repeat.

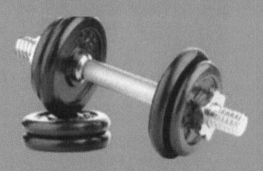

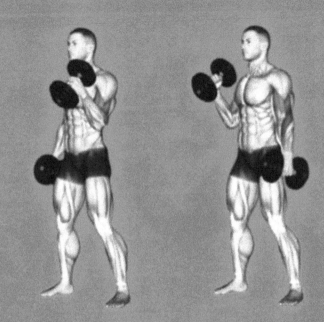

Hammer Bicep
Curl Exercise

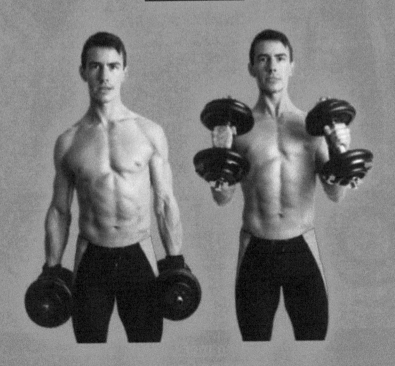

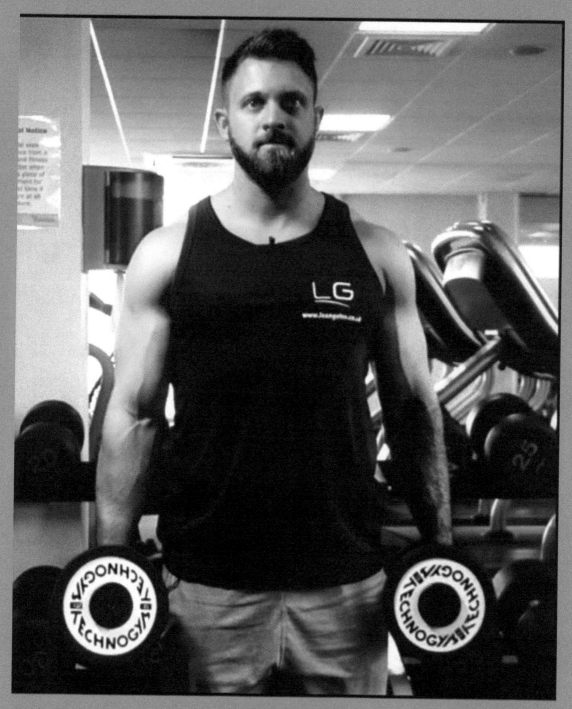

<u>Hammer Curl</u>
Starting Position

168

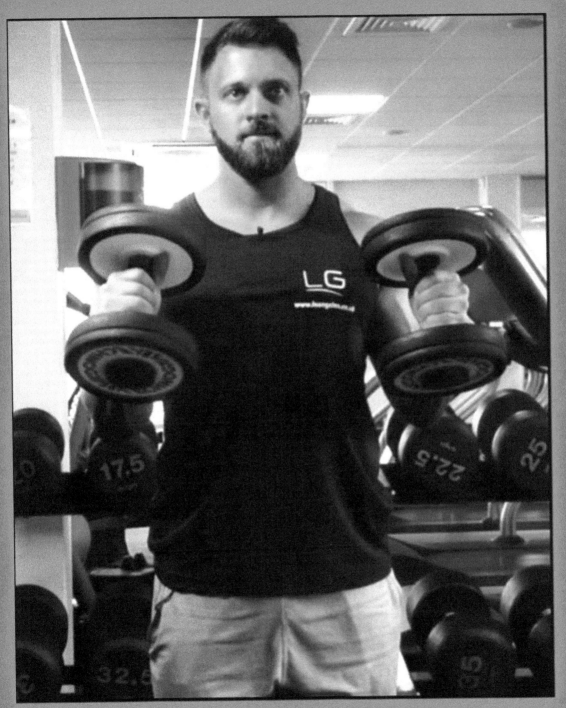

Hammer Curl
Finishing Position

CHIN-UPS

1. Grip the chin up bar with an **underhand grip** so that your palms are facing your body.

2. Ensure that your arms are a few inches apart so that they're in **line with your shoulders**.

3. Take a deep breath, keep your torso firm and **bring chest outwards slightly**.

4. Exhale as you use your upper arms to lift your body toward the bar, and stop when your chin is above the bar. Exhale whilst you're doing this.

5. **Only your arms should be doing the lifting work**. In other words, the torso should remain stationary and the forearms should do no other work other than hold the bar.

6. Hold in the top position for a second, inhale and return slowly back to the starting position.

7. Repeat.

Additional Tips

- Technically, the chin up, a bit like the pull up, is a great exercise for working out the back muscles [latissimus dorsi].

- As a general rule of thumb, however, the chin up (with an underhand grip) **places more emphasis on the biceps than the traditional wide grip pull up**.

- More emphasis is placed on the biceps directly the closer together the hands are (although the difference is minimal).

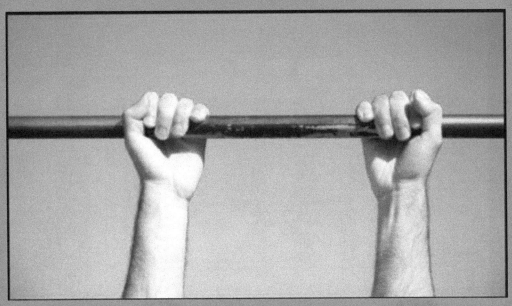

Figure 28:

Ensure an underhand grip so that palms are facing your body.

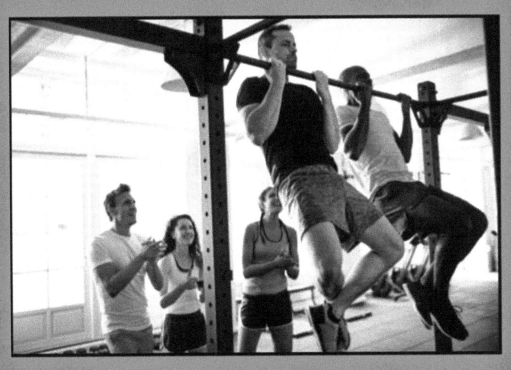

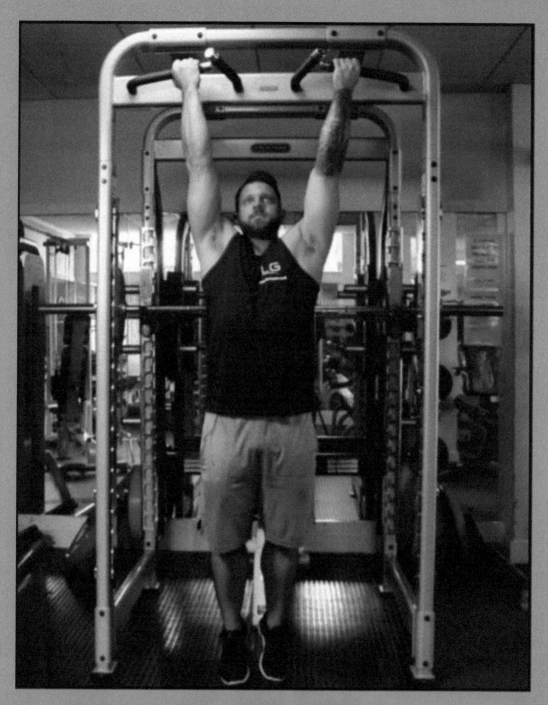

<u>Chin Up</u>
Starting Position

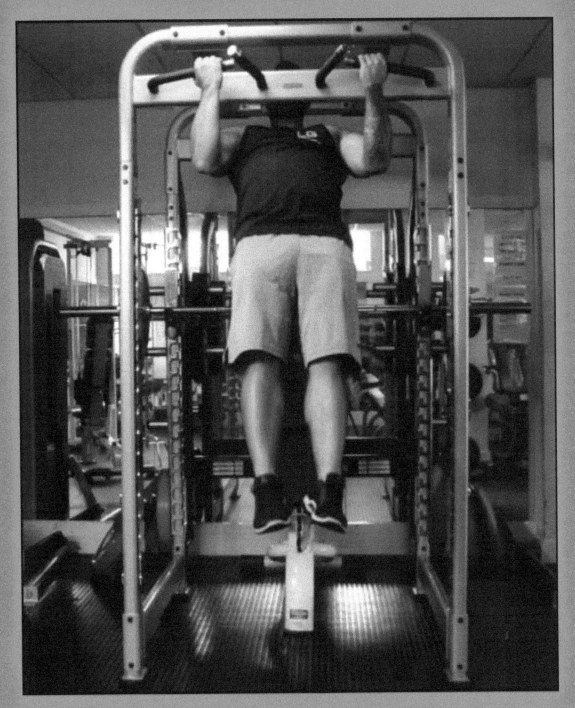

<u>Chin Up</u>
Finishing Position

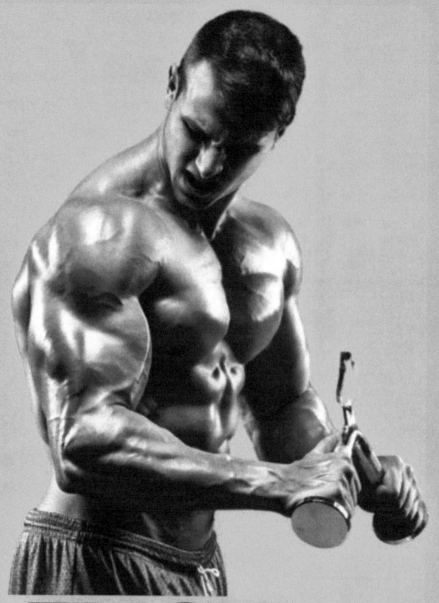

TRICEP
WORKOUTS

TRICEP WORKOUTS

CLOSE-GRIP BARBELL BENCH PRESS

SKULL CRUSHERS

TRICEP PUSHDOWN

DUMBBELL OVERHEAD TRICEP PRESS

DIPS

TRICEP MUSCLES

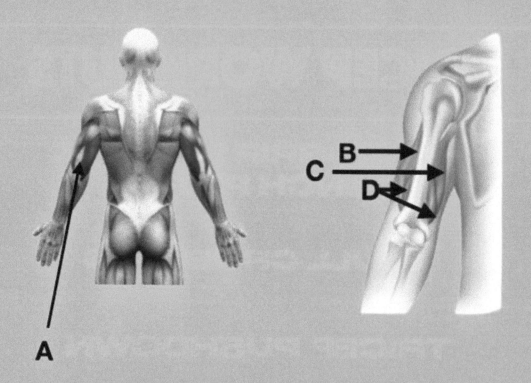

A = TRICEPS BRACHII
The triceps muscle has three heads, the long head, the lateral head and the medial head.

B = LATERAL HEAD
C = LONG HEAD
D = MEDIAL HEAD

TRICEP WORKOUTS

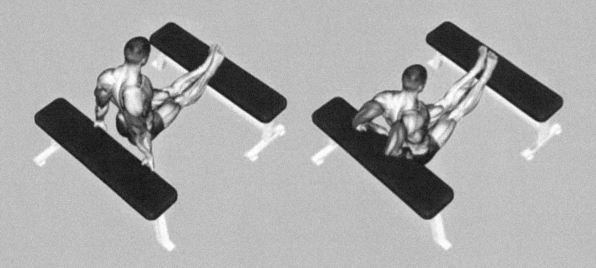

TRICEP WORKOUTS
Close-Grip Barbell Bench Press
Skull Crushers
Triceps Pushdown Dumbbell Overhead
Tricep Press
Dips

CLOSE-GRIP BARBELL BENCH PRESS

1. Select your weight and use a flat bench ideally, but you can use an incline as well.

2. Keep your feet flat on the floor and hold the barbell shoulder-width apart (hands should be 8-10 inches apart). **Do not hold the barbell any narrower** otherwise you'll put a tremendous amount of pressure on your elbow and wrist joints (Figure 29).

3. Keep torso tight and arc the back as you would for barbell chest press and **inhale** as you lift the bar.

4. Bring the bar downwards towards your upper torso/lower chest.

5. Keep shoulders in contact with bench (i.e., ensure they're not lifting up).

6. Keep elbows slightly flared out at a **30 degree flare** (i.e., do not keep too close to torso as this will create a lot of stress on your shoulder joints)

7. Don't touch the body but instead hold in this position for a second or so.

8. Exhale as you lift the bar Return to starting position and repeat.

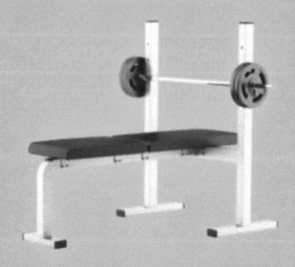

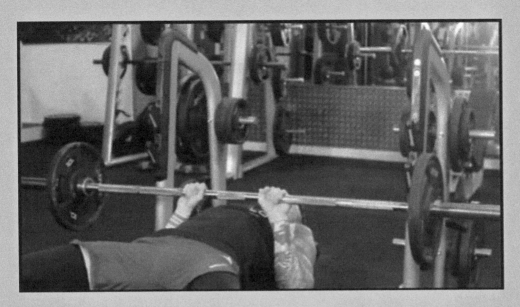

Close-Grip Barbell Press
Starting Position

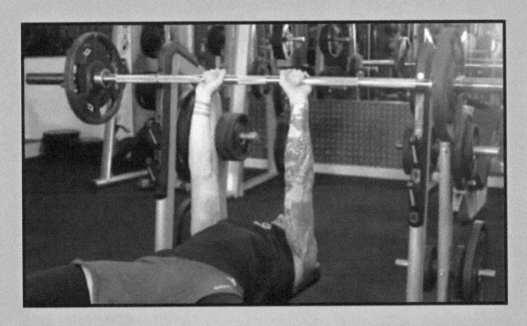

Close-Grip Barbell Press
Finishing Position

179

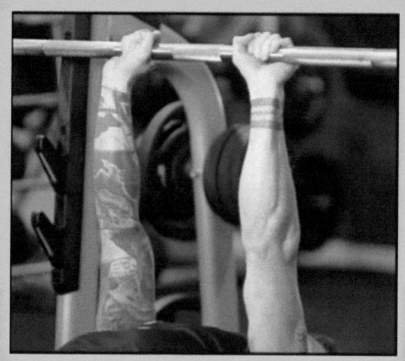

Figure 29:

*Hold The Barbell Shoulder-width so that
Hands are 8-10 Inches Apart.*

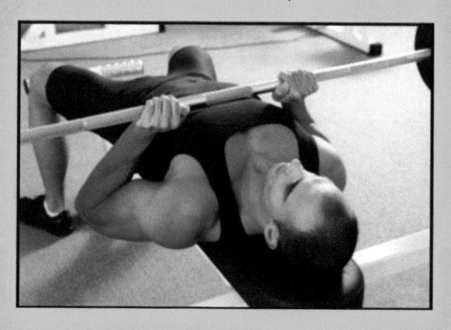

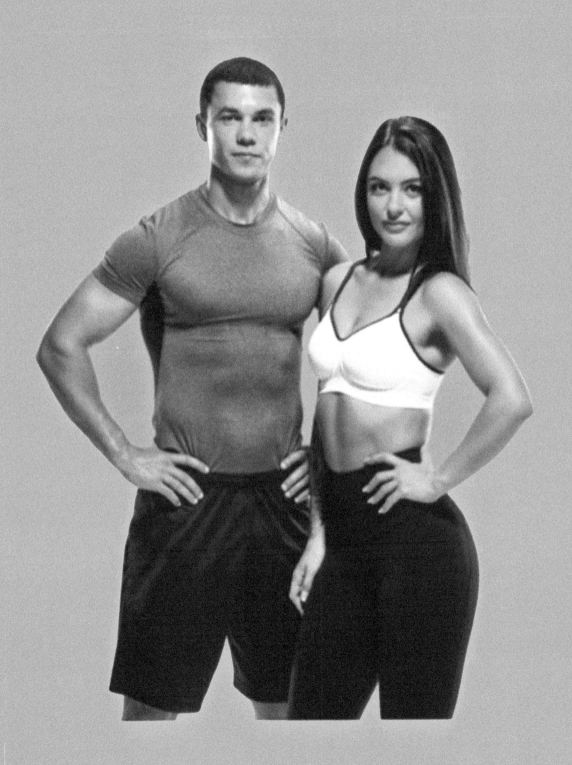

SKULL CRUSHERS

1. Select your weight and lay down on a flat bench ideally, but this can be done on an incline bench.

2. This exercise can be done with a barbell or dumbbell, but it's usually done with a **straight barbell or E-Z barbell**. In this case, we will be using a barbell.

3. Ensure feet are **firm on the floor** and torso engaged.

4. Lift barbell above your chest at just over thumb- to-thumb distance apart (Figure 30). Keep your arms firm and straight.

5. Then, in this position, squeeze the shoulder blades and trapezius muscles together and into the bench to increase stability.

6. Bring the barbell above your eyes/forehead. This will be your starting position.

7. Take a deep breath and exhale as you bring the barbell in a downwards arc.

8. As you do this, the only movement of the arms should be as it **rotates around your elbow**. In other words, avoid moving your upper arms back and forth from their position as you lower the weight (same applies to when you raise the weight back to the starting position).

9. Continue this downward and backward arc of motion towards the forehead (Figure 30) whilst maintaining tension within your triceps.

10. Return to starting position.

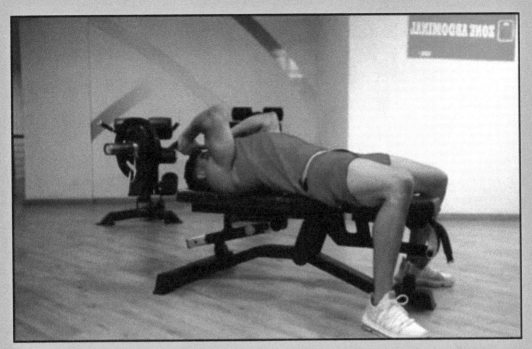

Conventional Skull Crusher - Starting Position

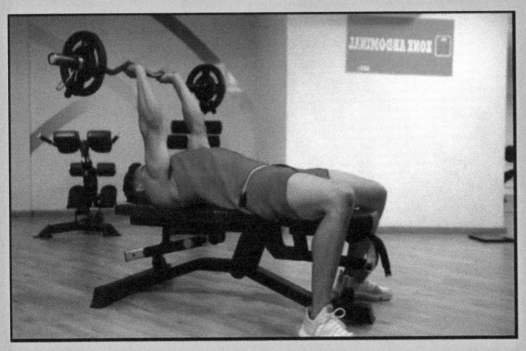

Conventional Skull Crusher - Finishing Position

183

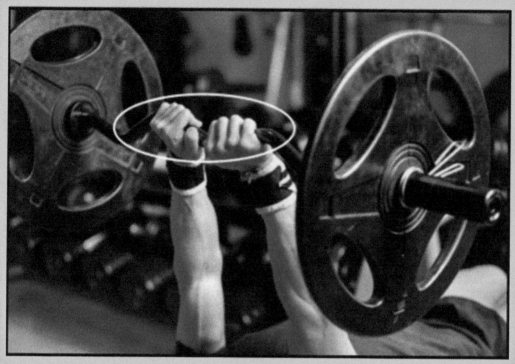

Figure 30:

*Lift barbell above your chest at just
over thumb- to-thumb distance apart*

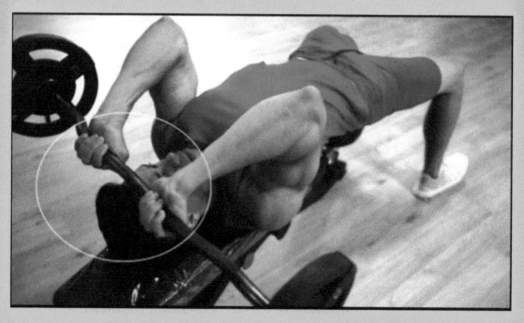

184

The 45-Degree Angle Version

- There are many ways to perform the skull-crusher exercise, but a **popular variation is the '45- degree angle' variation**. This involves:

  1. Placing your **upper arms above and behind your head at a 45-degree angle.**

  2. Then bring the bar in a **downward arc towards the bench** so that the bar goes behind the head and touches/almost touches the bench.

- The advantage of the 45-degree variation is that you get better tricep involvement due to a **greater range of movement**. Many personal trainers and bodybuilders prefer this version of the skull-crusher for this reason. In addition, the 45-degree angle **works against gravity** which adds more tension to the movement.

- Another advantage of the '45-degree/back of the head' version is that it tends to **take a lot of tension away from the elbow-region** proving to be much kinder to your elbows.

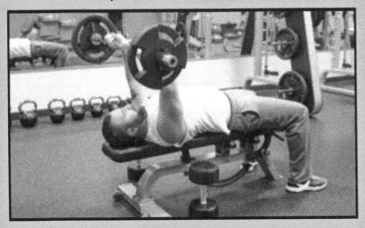

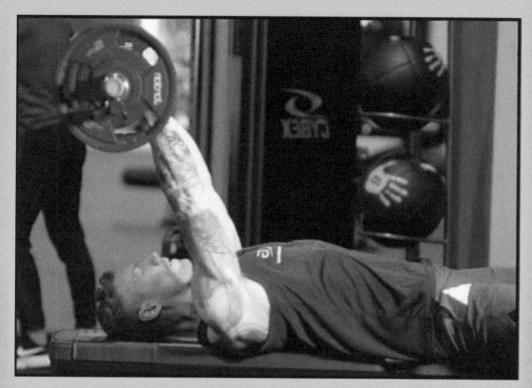

Skull-Crushers
45-Degree Version

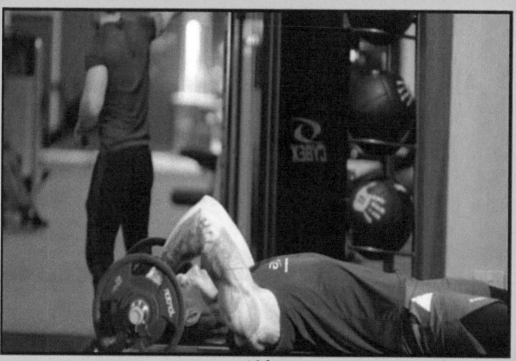

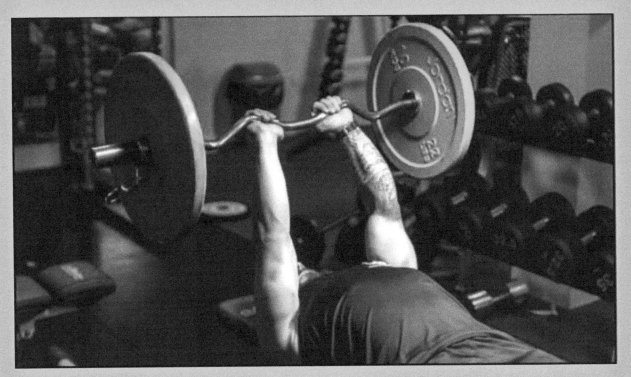

Skull-Crushers
45-Degree Version

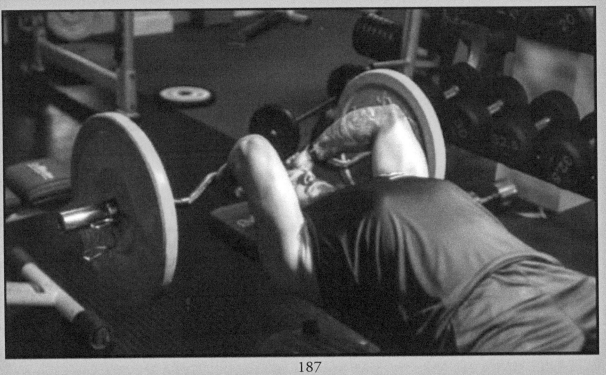

DUMBBELL OVERHEAD TRICEP PRESS

1. Ideally find a seat with back support.

2. Grab your dumbbell, sit down and **place behind your shoulders.**

3. Ensure **feet are flat on the ground and torso is firm.**

4. When holding the dumbbell, make sure you're using **both hands palms up** towards the ceiling so that they're pressing along the inner aspect of the outer dumbbell plate with your thumbs around it.

5. **Straighten** your arms with the weight behind your head.

6. From this position, **move and rotate your arms and dumbbell forwards sightly until it's above your head**. If you're sitting in front of a mirror, the outer disc should be facing the mirror. This will be your **starting position**.

7. Inhale and bring dumbbell **downwards behind your head** whilst keeping the rest of your body firm and your upper arms stationary. Keep your elbows tucked in and close to your body as you do this.

8. Continue this movement until your **biceps and forearms touch.**

9. **Return** to starting position and repeat.

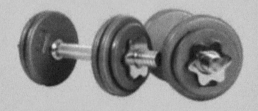

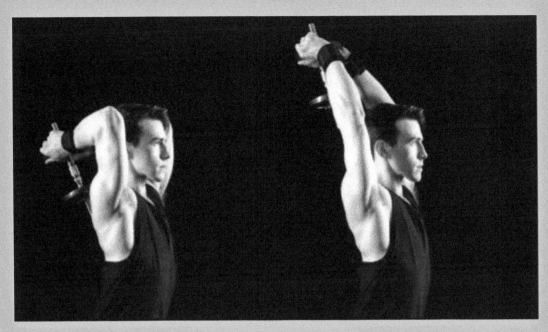

Dumbbell-Overhead

Tricep Press

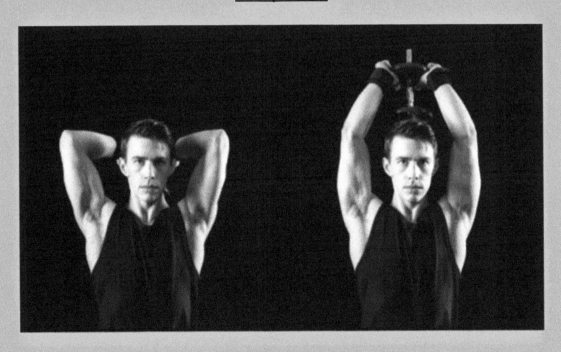

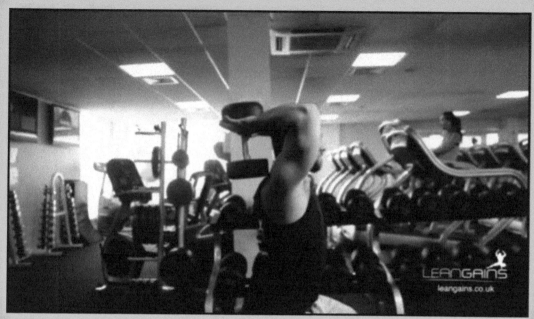

Dumbbell-Overhead Tricep Press
(Without Back-Support)
Starting Position

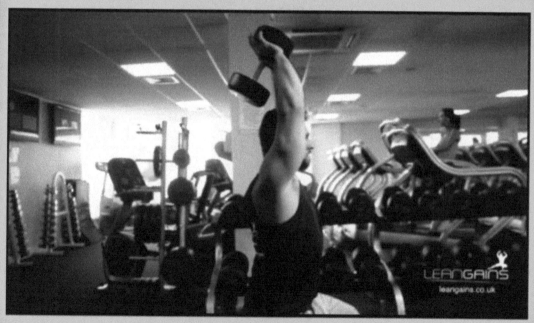

Dumbbell-Overhead Tricep Press
(Without Back-Support)
Finishing Position

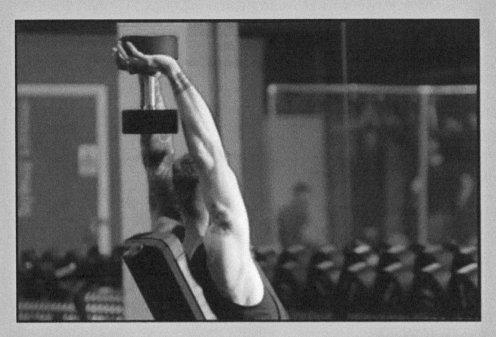

<u>Dumbbell-Overhead Tricep Press</u>
(With Back-Support)
Starting Position

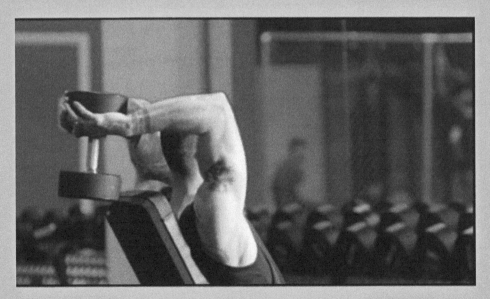

<u>Dumbbell-Overhead Tricep Press</u>
(With Back-Support)
Finishing Position

191

TRICEP PUSHDOWN

1. Attach a bar (straight/angled) to the machine and select weight.

2. Attach a bar to the machine. I would suggest using the rope, but there are many bars you can use such as:

   - Straight Bar (Figure 31),

   - Rope (Figure 32),

   - V-Bar (Figure 33).

3. Grab rope/bar at **shoulder-width** with an **overhand grip** (palms facing downwards).

4. **Stand upright with torso firm** and lean forwards very slightly.

5. **Keep your feet together** with a slight bend in your knees.

6. Make sure that your **elbows are in front of your hips** at all times.

7. Bring the **rope/bar down until arms are straight**, and then return slowly until forearms are **just over 90 degrees to the floor**. The top of the bar should be level with your **lower chest.**

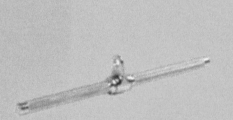 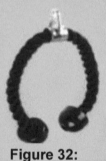 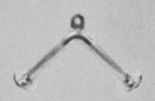

Figure 31:
Straight Bar.

Figure 32:
Rope.

Figure 33:
V-Bar.

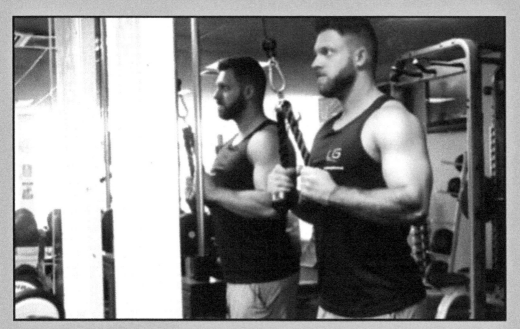

Tricep Pushdown - Starting Position

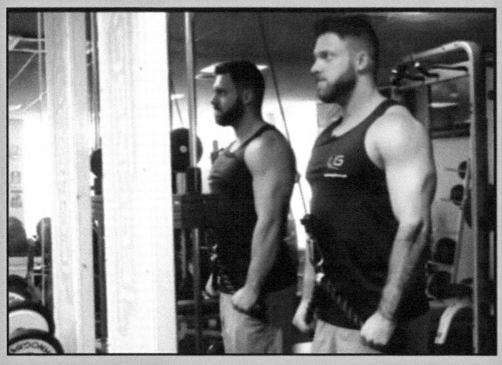

Tricep Pushdown - Finishing Position

DIPS

- **Dips are great for both chest and triceps**. However, we can position ourselves to **slightly** favour one over the other.

- In this variation, we are targeting the triceps more. **The main difference is how we position our elbows** which are as close to your body as possible.

1. **Grab the grip hard and squeeze firmly**. Your hands should be under your shoulders and close to your body.

2. **Balance yourself with straight arms** and locked elbows as your start position.

3. **Raise your chest** and keep your **shoulders back** (i.e., don't roll them forward).

4. **Lower your body by bending your arms** and, unlike with the chest variation whereby you're leaning forward slightly; for your triceps, you want to **keep your head and chest up**. You also want to **ensure your elbows are next to your torso throughout the movement**. Keep your torso tight.

5. Keep your **legs slightly bent** and/or cross your feet.

6. The 'end-position' should be when your **shoulders are below your elbows.**

7. Raise up by straightening arms and keeping everything else firm.

8. At the top position, **bring chest outwards** and straighten arms whilst maintaining tension within triceps.

9. Repeat.

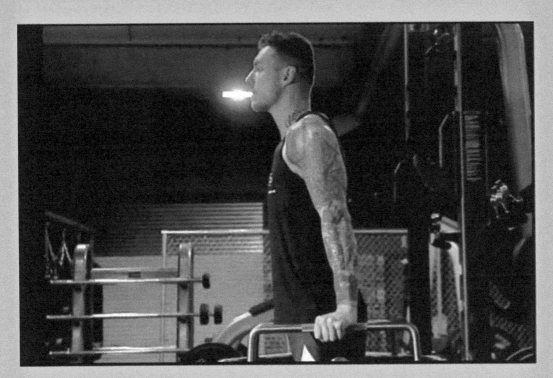

Dips - Starting Position

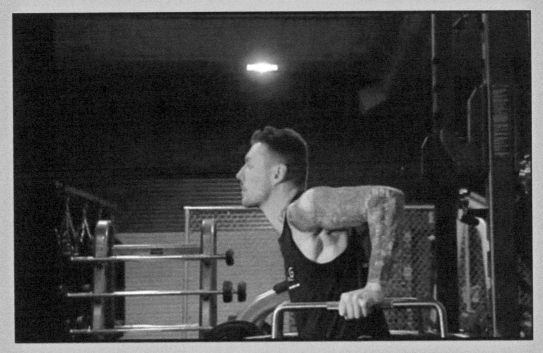

Dips - Finishing Position

An Alternative Version

- A very popular alternative to the conventional 'dip' exercise is to do them using 1 or 2 chairs/benches. If you're using a chair, make sure it's stable so you don't slip.

1. Sit on a chair or bench with hands just outside of the hips.

2. You can choose to keep your knees bent if you're new to this exercise. However, straightening the legs will make this exercise more challenging.

3. Bring the hips close to the bench/chair and grab the edge of it so that your palms are facing away from your body.

4. Then proceed to lifting yourself up onto your hands until your arms are straight.

5. Bend the elbows and lower down to about 90 degrees so that your elbows are pointing behind you (Figure 34).

6. Keep the shoulders down and the core/abs engaged.

Additional Tips

- **Remember to keep your hips close to the chair or bench** to avoid straining the shoulders. Make sure you keep the shoulders down and away from the ears.

- **You can use 2 benches if you like** (Figure 35). This makes the exercise more challenging. Basically, it's the same as the above routine, but you need to lift your feet so that your heels are resting on the other bench and your legs are straight. If you're with a friend, you can increase the difficulty by getting him/her to place a weight on your quads (thighs) but if you choose to do this, then be careful and keep your core tight to reduce risk of back injury.

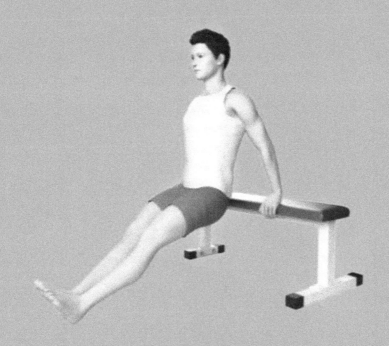

Dips - Starting Position

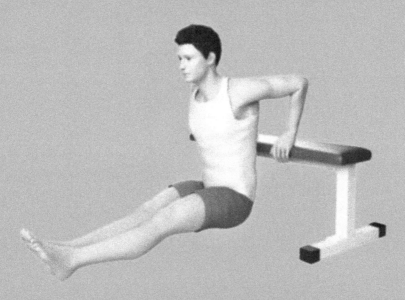

Dips - Finishing Position

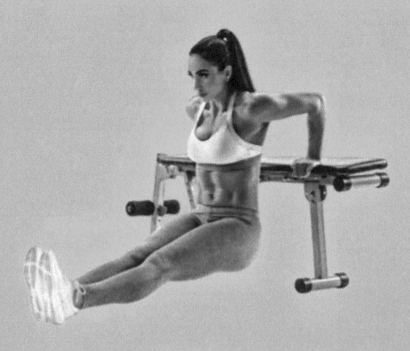

Figure 34:
*Bend your elbows and lower down to about 90 degrees.
Elbows should be pointing behind you.*

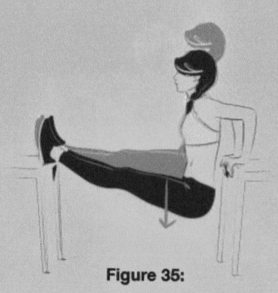

Figure 35:

*If you use 2 benches, make sure your legs are straight. If you're training with
a friend, you can get him/her to place some weights onto your quads to make
this exercise more challenging.*

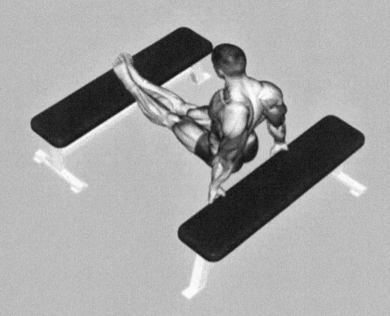

Dips - Starting Position

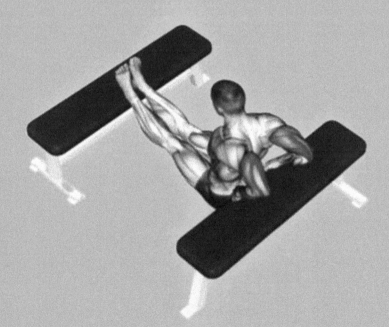

Dips - Finishing Position

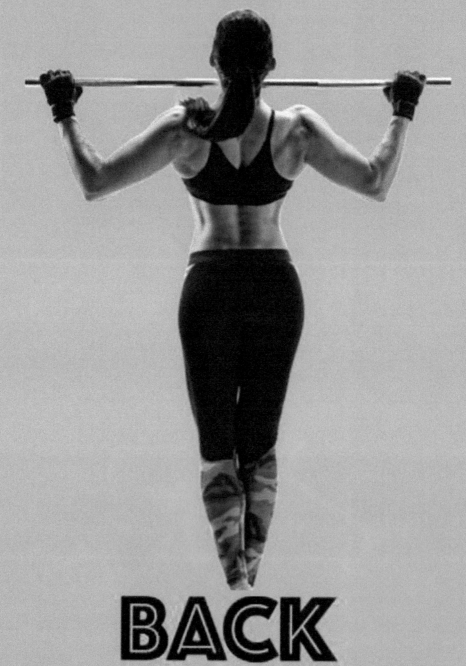

BACK WORKOUTS

BACK WORKOUTS

BARBELL DEADLIFT

WIDE-GRIP PULL-UP

BARBELL & T-BAR ROW

ONE-ARM DUMBBELL ROW

LAT PULLDOWN

BARBELL SHRUG

DUMBBELL SHRUG

HYPEREXTENSION

UPPER BACK MUSCLES

(TRAPS AND LATS)

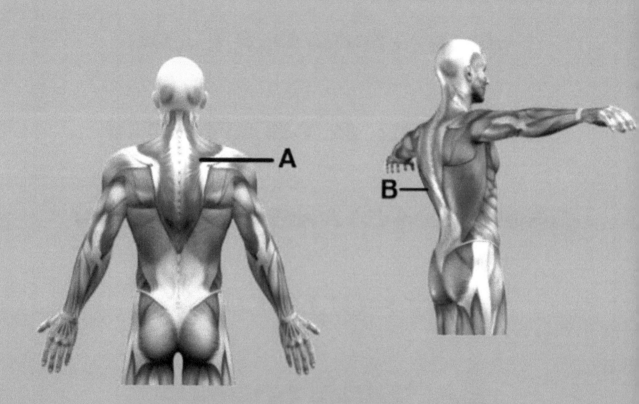

A = TRAPEZIUS (TRAPS)

B = LATISSIMUS DORSI (LATS)

UPPER BACK WORKOUTS

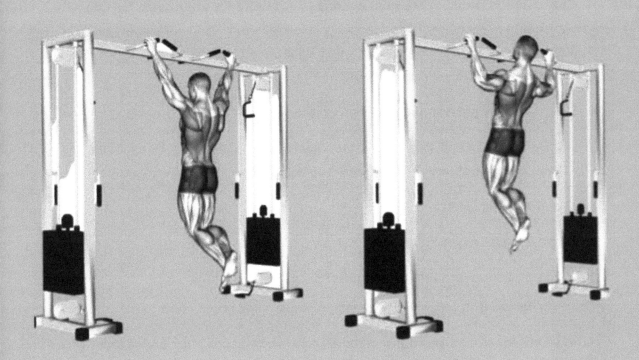

ENTIRE BACK	UPPER BACK	TRAPS
Barbell Deadlift	Wide Grip Pull-Ups	Shrug
	Shrugs	
Wide Grip Pull-Ups	Lat Pulldowns	
One-Arm Dumbbell Row	Barbell/T-Bar Row	
Barbell/T-Bar Row	One-Arm Dumbbell Row	

BARBELL DEADLIFT

- **The 'deadlift' is one of the best exercises out there for your back**, but can cause severe injury if not done properly. If you're new to this, make sure (as with all exercises) that you start off with a light weight and ensure you have perfect form before increasing weight.

1. Select your weight and **place barbell on the floor**.

2. Approach the bar until the **bar is 1-inch away (in front of) your shins**. The **laces on your trainers should be in front of the bar**.

3. Stand hip-width apart.

4. There are 2 ways you can grip the bar:

    1) **Double-overhand grip** (Figure 36).

    2) **Mixed-grip** (one overhand and one underhand grip (Figure 37)).

5. Hold the bar around **shoulder-width**. Ensure you're gripping the bar so that your hands are wider than your legs.

6. As you go down to lift the bar, your **shins should almost touch the bar** (Figure 38).

7. To avoid lumbar injury, once you've gripped the bar, **bring your hips down and your chest up** (Figure 39). Ensure torso is tight and that **there's an arc in your lower back**.

8. The lift consists of 2 movements (Figure 40 and 41):

    1) **Leg Exercise** - Lifting barbell to the knees.

    2) **Back Exercise** - Lifting barbell to the torso.

9. To lift the barbell to the knees, take a deep breath in and exhale as you lift the bar. **Make sure you're pressing your feet/heels** into the ground as you do this.

10. The bar should be in **close proximity to your shins** as you lift.

11. Once the bar reaches the knees, your **back muscles will kick in after that**.

12. Continue lifting the bar so that it's in **close proximity to your thighs**. Drive through with the hips until your **legs are straight** at which point you can **lock your hips and knees**. Do not shrug or lean backwards at this position.

13. **Return the weight by unlocking your knees and hips, and moving the weight down your thighs, along a downward arc of closure, and then bend the knees as you return the weight to the floor.**

14. Return the weight to the floor at **almost free-fall speed** (as if you're dropping the barbell to the floor) but hold the barbell tight as you do this. The barbell deadlift is similar to the Pendlay Row in this regard.

15. Repeat.

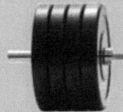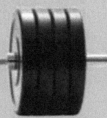

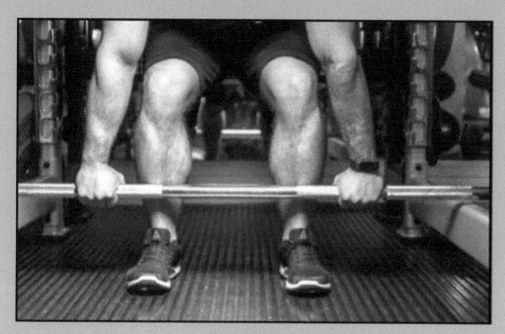

Figure 36:
Double Overhand Grip.

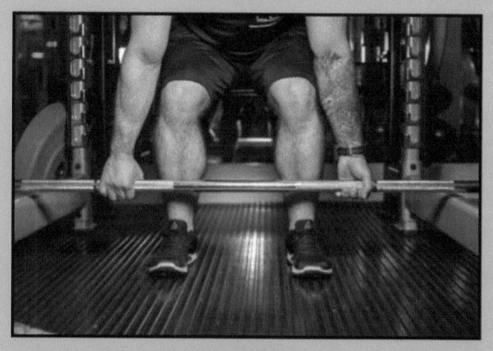

Figure 37:
The 'Mixed' Grip.
206

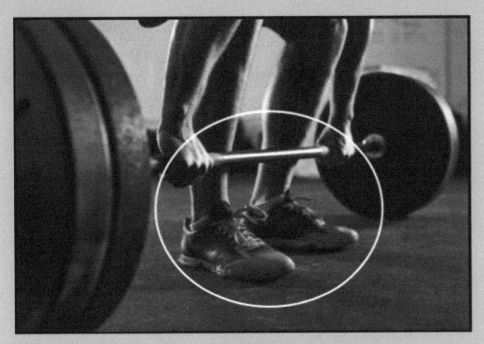

Figure 38:
*Your Shins Should Almost Touch the Bar so bar is
Positioned over Mid-Foot Region.*

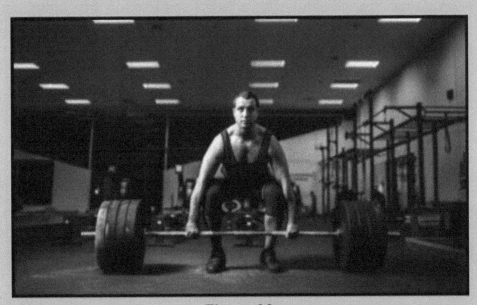

Figure 39:
Bring Your Hips Down and Your Chest Up.

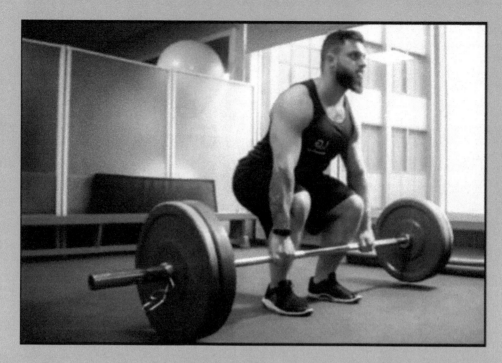

Barbell Deadlift Deadlift - Starting Position

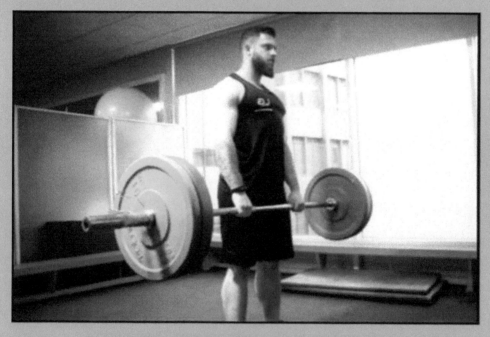

Barbell Deadlift Deadlift - Finishing Position

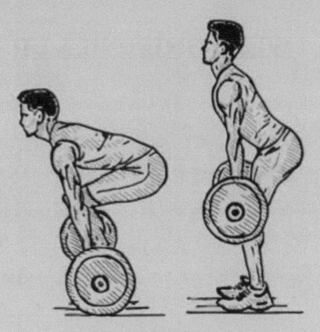

Figure 40:
First Part of the 'Deadlift Movement' Involves
Lifting Barbell to the Knees from the Floor.
Depress Hip and Lift Chest.

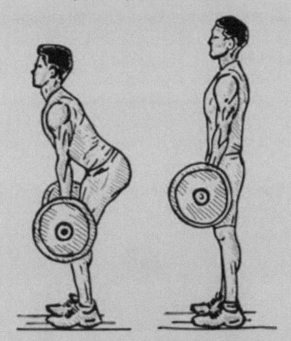

Figure 41:
Second Part of the 'Deadlift Movement' Involves
Lifting Barbell to the Torso from the Knees

<u>WIDE GRIP PULL UP</u>

1. Use a pronated (palms facing floor) and wide grip (slightly wider than shoulder width) on a pull-up bar.

2. Elevate the chest, take a deep breath and squeeze the glutes and abs.

3. **Depress the shoulder blades** whilst pulling the **elbows towards the floor**. This way, you're compressing your lats.

4. **Pull your chin towards the bar** until the lats are fully contracted. This should be done in a vertical motion (i.e., **no swinging**).

<u>Useful Tips</u>

- Use the **'assisted' wide-grip pull up machine** if you're having difficulty doing the pull-up using the bar alone. Alternatively, use the **'lat pulldown' machine.**

- Aim for a **full range of motion**.

- Keep a neutral head position (looking straight ahead or slightly up).

- **Crossing your legs is optional**, but will help stabilise your body during the lift.

- **Uncrossing your legs** will engage your core a lot more.

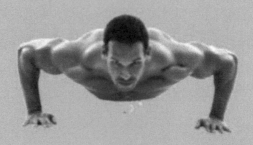

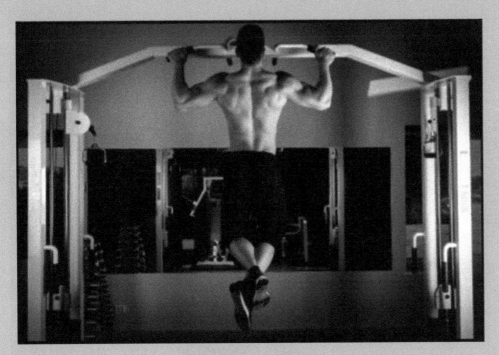

Wide-Grip Pull Up
Crossed Legs

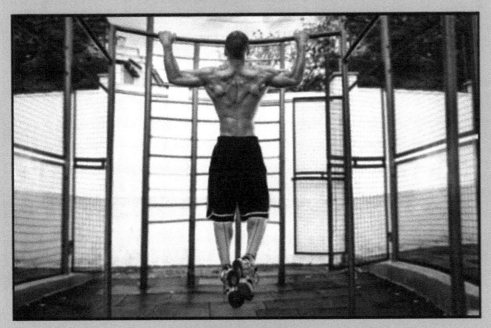

Wide-Grip Pull Up
Un-Crossed Legs

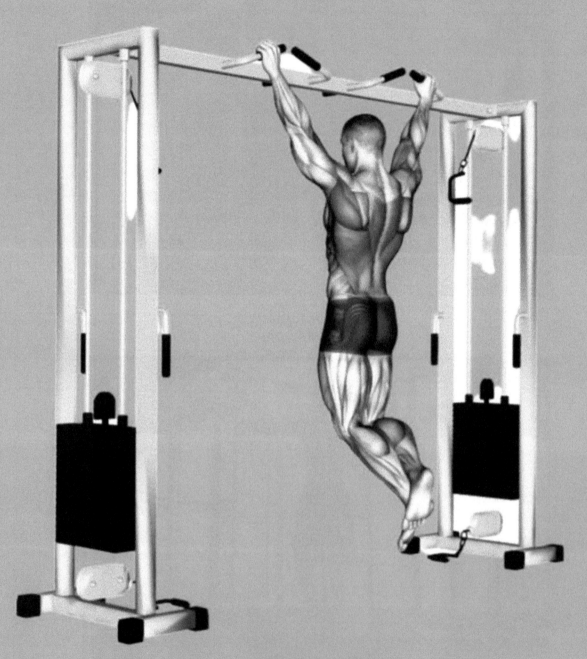

<u>Wide-Grip Pull Up</u>
Starting Position

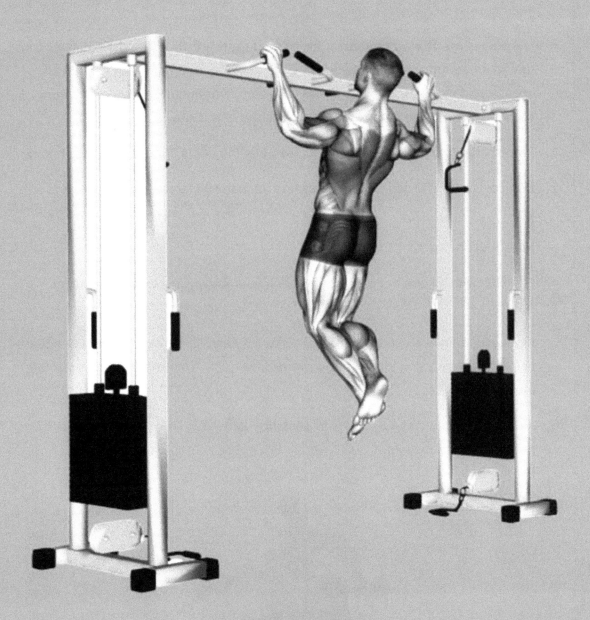

<u>Wide-Grip Pull Up</u>
Finishing Position

213

BARBELL ROW

- The barbell row is **very similar** to the **barbell rear-delt row**. The main difference is that when performing the 'rear-delt row' (or "Pendlay Row"), the bar is lifted to chest level to engage the deltoid muscles more, **whereas here, we're bringing the bar towards the abs so as to engage the lats more.**

1. Place barbell in a rack at a low position so that the bar is knee-level or just below.

2. Bend over at 45-60 degree angle towards the bar with knees slightly bent and firm torso.

3. Keep feet shoulder-width apart.

4. Grab bar with an overhand grip just wide of your knees (just outside shoulder width).

5. Keep your elbows close to your body, torso tight and lift bar from just under knee position upwards along thigh path towards lower abs. **This will engage your lats mainly.**

6. Alternatively, to train your traps and posterior delts, then lift bar towards your lower chest/upper abs instead.

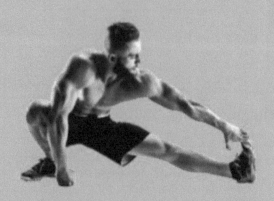

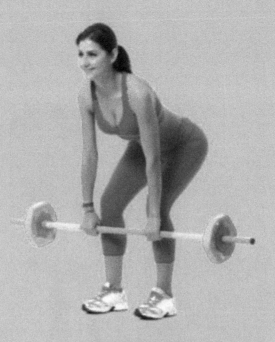

Barbell Row
Starting Position

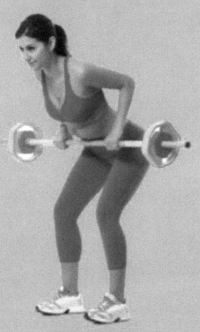

Barbell Row
Finishing Position

215

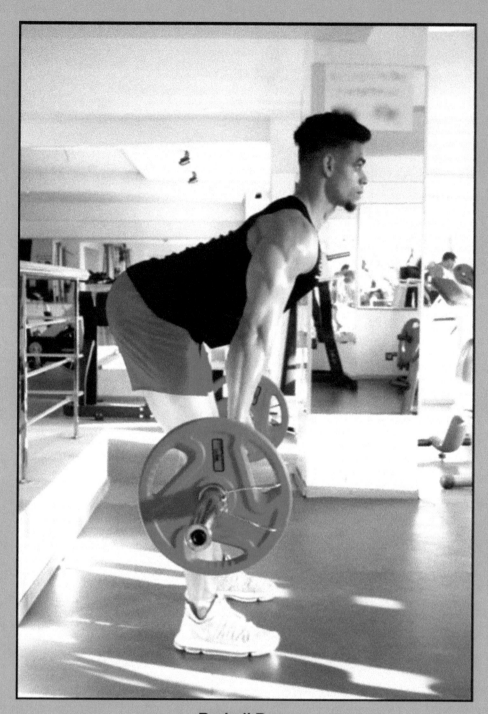

Barbell Row
Starting Position

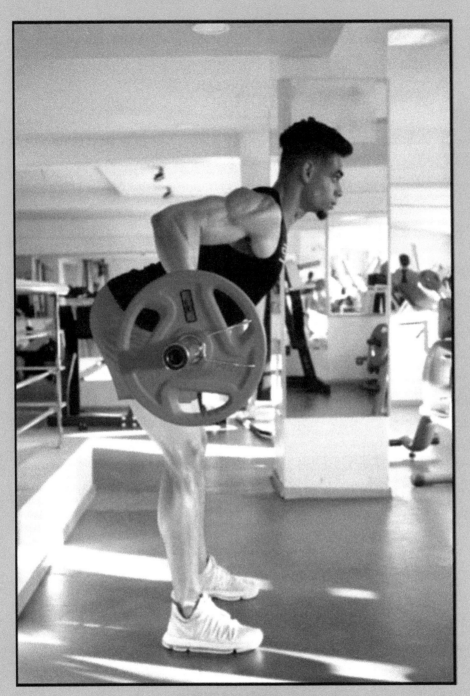

<u>Barbell Row</u>
Finishing Position

ONE-ARM DUMBBELL ROW

1. Grab a bench and a dumbbell.

2. If you're **training your right arm**, position your **left shin onto one end of the bench** and your **left hand palms down flat** on the other side (Figure 42). Alternatively, use the left hand to grip the other end of the bench at the end.

3. Place your right leg straight on the floor.

4. Bend your torso forward from the waist and chest slightly upright until your upper body is parallel to the floor.

5. Your starting position is when the dumbbell is held with arms straight but not fully extended so that there's a slight bend in the elbows.

6. Make sure the rest of the body is stationary and back is parallel to the floor whilst lifting the dumbbell.

7. As you lift your dumbbell, keep your wrists straight and lift the dumbbell towards your armpits keeping the elbows close to the body at all times (Figure 43).

8. Do the same on the other side for your left arm.

Useful Tips

Ensure you engage your back once you reach the contracted position at the top of the movement. The majority of the force should be coming from your back and not your hands.

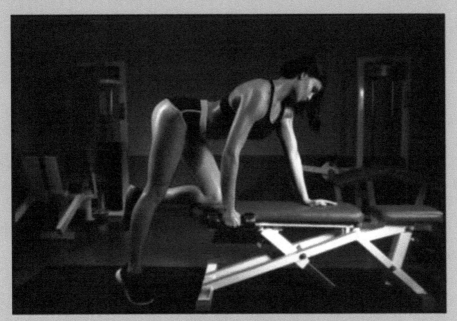

Figure 42:
*Position your left shin onto one end of the bench and
your left hand palms down flat on the other side.*

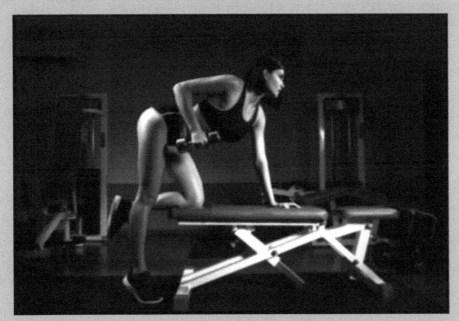

Figure 43:
*Ensure the rest of the body is **stationary** and back is parallel
to the floor whilst lifting the dumbbell.*

219

LAT PULLDOWNS

• The 'lat pulldown' is a **good alternative** for those who struggle doing lat pull-ups.

1. Sit down in a 'lat pulldown' machine and select weight.

2. Get a wide bar and attach to the top pulley. Make sure you adjust the **knee pad to fit your height**. These pads prevent your body from moving during the exercise.

3. Grab the bar with a **wide-grip (slightly wider than shoulder-width)** and **palms facing downwards.**

4. Bring your body (i.e., torso) back slightly (**around 30 degrees**), create a **curvature on your lower back and stick your chest out.**

5. Inhale and keep your **elbows slightly in front of your body**, exhale as you **pull down in line with your hips** in a straight line.

6. **Keep your chest tall** as you bring the bar to your chest (Figure 44). Never bring the bar behind your neck.

7. Focus more on **using your lats to pull the weight as opposed to your biceps** (this takes some practice in the beginning). One way of helping you do this is if you **place your thumb on top of the bar,** as opposed to underneath it, as you're pulling it down.

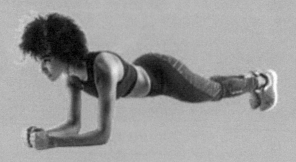

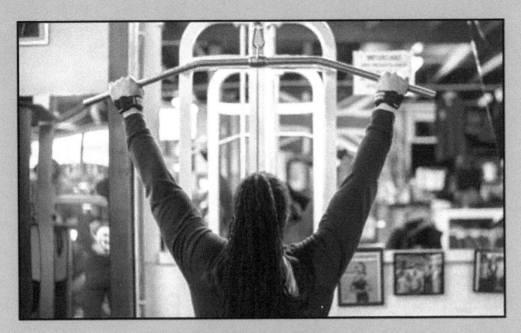

Wide-Grip Lateral Pulldown
Starting Position

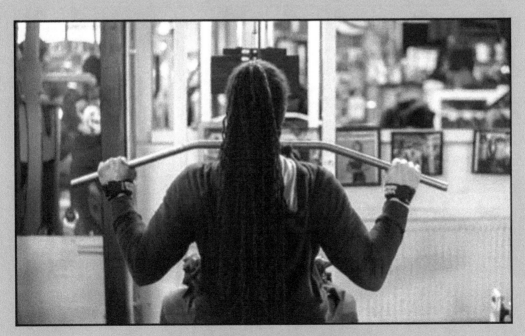

Wide-Grip Lateral Pulldown
Finishing Position

221

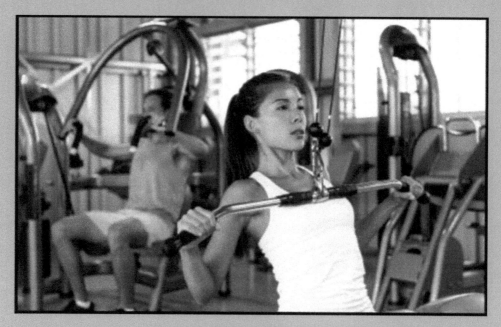

Figure 44:

Keep Your Chest Tall as you bring the bar to your chest.

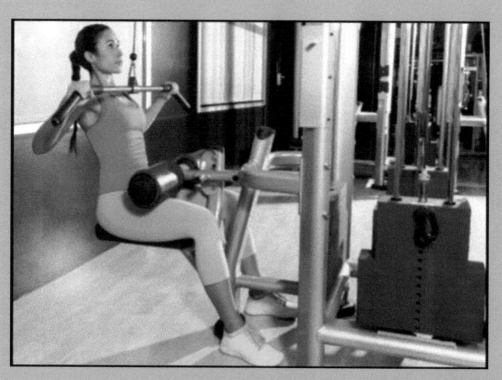

BARBELL SHRUG

1. Place barbell in a rack at a low position so that the bar is around **knee-level**.

2. Select desired weight.

3. Ensure **hands are slightly wider than shoulder- width apart** (your little finger should be aligned to the smooth line on the bar), and hold the barbell with a pronated grip (palms facing thighs).

4. **Inhale as you lift**, stick your chest out and arch your back ensuring a tight torso.

5. Ensure a **sight bend in your knees,** and lift up the weight as you exhale.

6. Raise your shoulders as far as you can whilst maintaining a straight arm (i.e., don't use your biceps to lift). Shrug your shoulders as you lift.

7. Return to starting position and repeat.

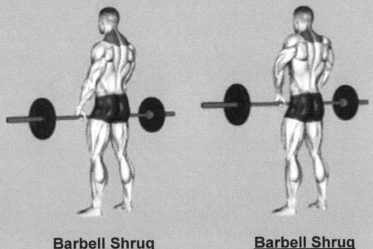

Barbell Shrug
Starting Position

Barbell Shrug
Finishing Position

DUMBBELL SHRUG

1. Pick up a pair of dumbbells.

2. Stand shoulder-width apart.

3. Ensure tight torso and chest outwards.

4. **Retract** your shoulder blades.

5. Elevate your shoulders **upwards and backwards** until your traps are fully contracted.

6. Return to starting position and repeat.

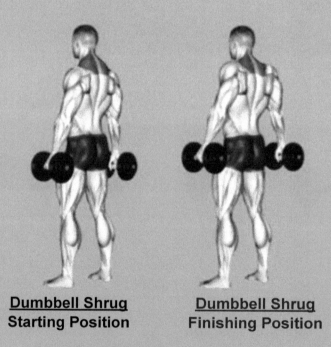

**Dumbbell Shrug
Starting Position**

**Dumbbell Shrug
Finishing Position**

T-BAR ROW

1. Use a **T-bar holder** (Figure 45) to position one end of a barbell in place (most gyms should have a T-bar holder).

2. **Load the other side of the bar** with your desired weight.

3. Take a '**Double-D row handle'/V-bar** (Figure 46 and Figure 47) and place it around the **underside of the bar at the inner end** where the weight is loaded.

4. Stand with a **wide-stance (slightly wider than shoulder-width)** with your hips back and chest up until you're **45 degree angle to the floor** (Figure 48).

5. Ensure your core is tight, your glutes are engaged, and your **back is slightly arched** so as to maintain a n**eutral spine. Your arms should be extended**. This is your **starting position**.

6. Take a deep breath and **pull the weight towards your chest**. As you do so, drive your elbows back and **squeeze your shoulder blades together** (as if using them to squeeze a tennis ball).

7. Pause for a second before returning to the start position.

Useful Tips

- Make sure you maintain your posture throughout and **never round your back** at any point.

- Try not to jerk the movement. Keep the movement as smooth and controlled as possible (this can be difficult when working with heavy weights).

- I've said this already, but **ensure your glutes are engaged throughout the entire movement** to prevent lower back/lumbar injury. **Pressing into the floor with your heals** helps maintain gluteal muscle engagement.

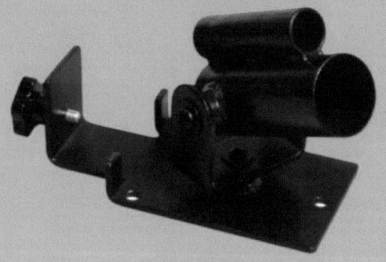

Figure 45:
T-Bar Holder

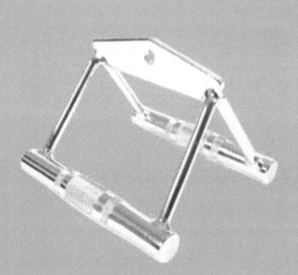

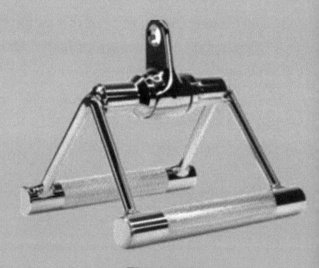

Figure 47:
Double-D Row Handle

Figure 46:
V-Bar

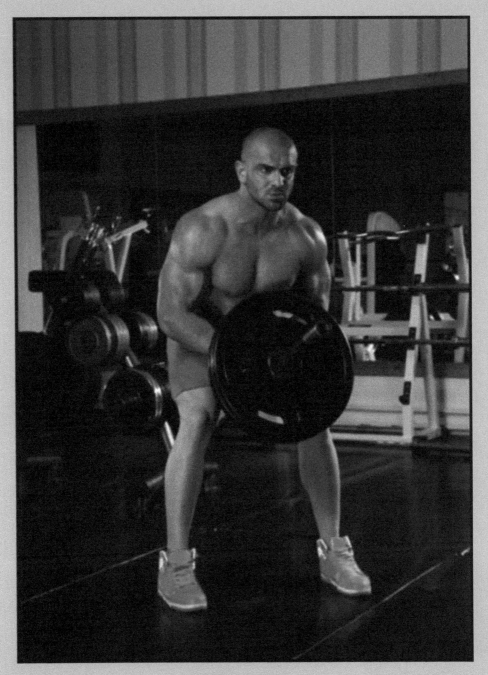

Figure 48:
Make Sure Chest (Upper Body)
Is 45 Degrees to the Floor.

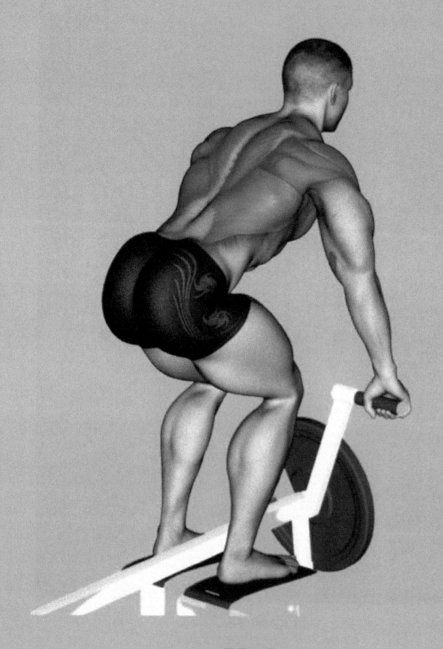

T-Bar Row
Starting Position

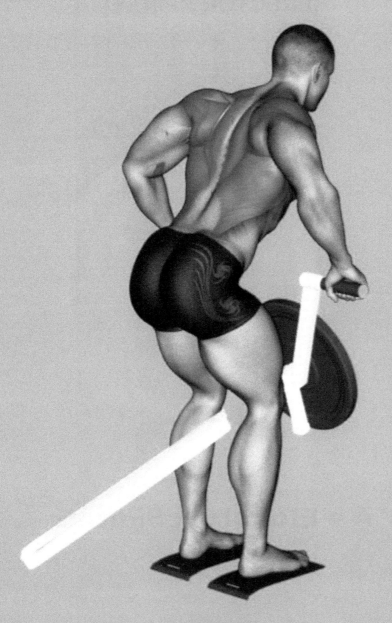

T-Bar Row
Finishing Position

LOWER BACK MUSCLES

(ERECTOR SPINAE)

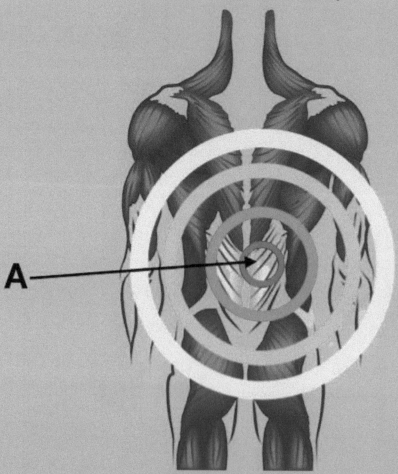

A

A = ERECTOR SPINAE

LOWER BACK WORKOUTS

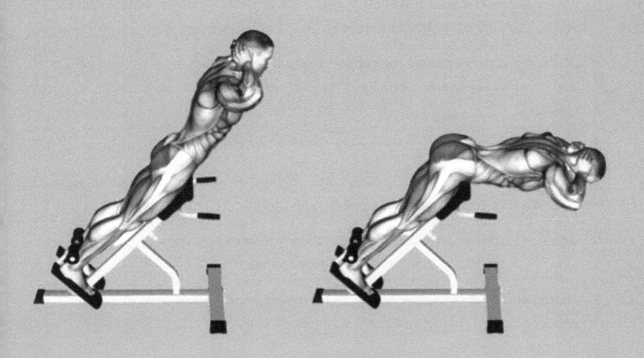

```
LOWER BACK

Barbell Deadlift

Hyperextension
```

HYPEREXTENSION

1. Find a '**back extension' machine** (Figure 49) and position yourself so that your **ankles are supported by the footpads**.

2. Adjust the **upper pad until your upper thighs lie flat across the wide pad** (Figure 50). This should leave enough room for you to bend at the waist without any restriction.

3. Keep **torso tight and chest outwards**.

4. **Cross your arms in front of your chest or place them behind your head** (Figure 51 & 52). If you're using a weight, hold it in front of you.

5. Inhale and bend forward until you **feel a stretch in your hamstrings**. Avoid rounding of the back-this means you've gone too low.

6. **Raise your torso back to starting position until your body is straight (as in plank position)**. There's no need to go higher than this.

Useful Tips

• You can either do this exercise using your **body only or by holding a weight**.

• If you're going to use a weight, hold the weight with **both hands in front of your chest** throughout the movement.

• Another variation of this exercise is the '**superman hyperextension.**' Here, instead of crossing your arms or placing them behind your head, you're keeping them **straight down towards the floor in your down position and raising them upwards as you come up**. This creates more tension on your lower back making the exercise **harder** than the conventional hyperextension.

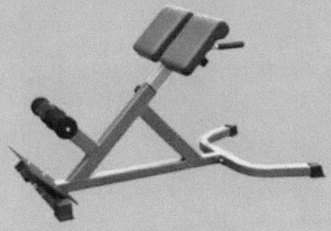

Figure 49:
'Back Extension' Machine.

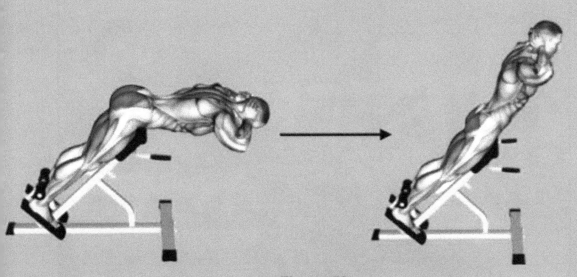

Figure 50:
'Upper Thighs Should Lie Across the Upper Wide Pad.

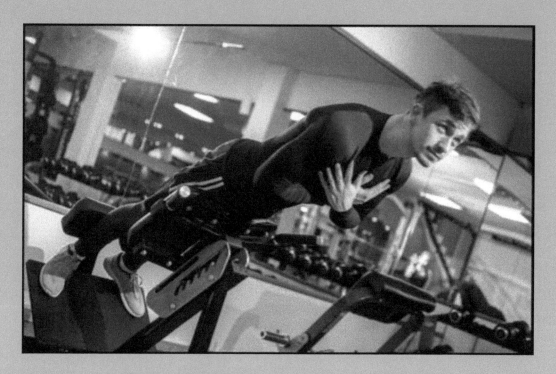

Figure 51: *Hyperextension with Crossed Hands*

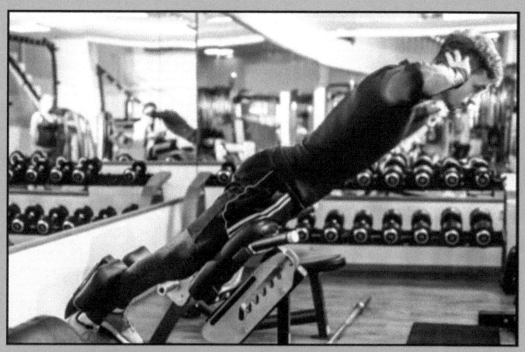

Figure 52: *Hyperextension with Hands on Head.*

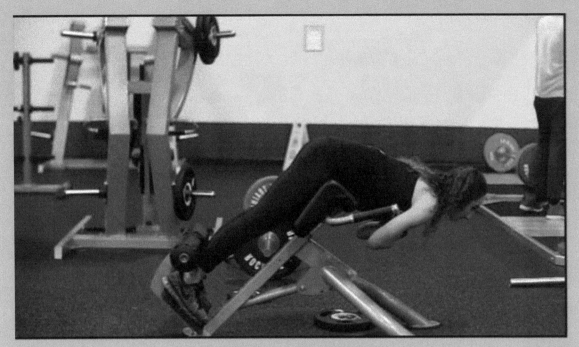

Hyperextension - Starting Position

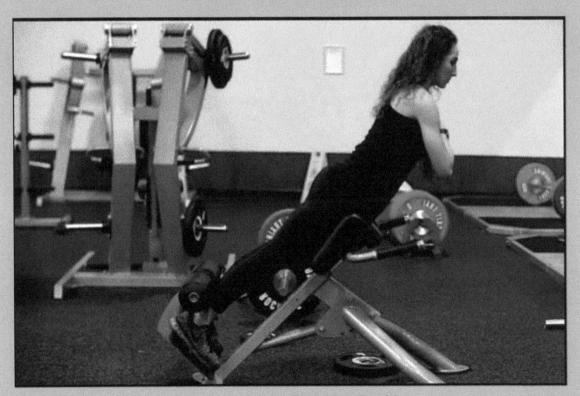

Hyperextension - Finishing Position

235

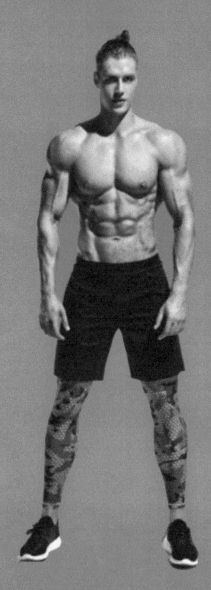

ABDOMINAL WORKOUTS

AB WORKOUTS

CABLE CRUNCHES

HANGING KNEE/LEG RAISES

CAPTAIN CHAIR LEG RAISES

AB ROLLER

AIR BICYCLES

DECLINE CRUNCH

ABDOMINAL MUSCLES

(VISIBLE ABDOMINAL MUSCLES)

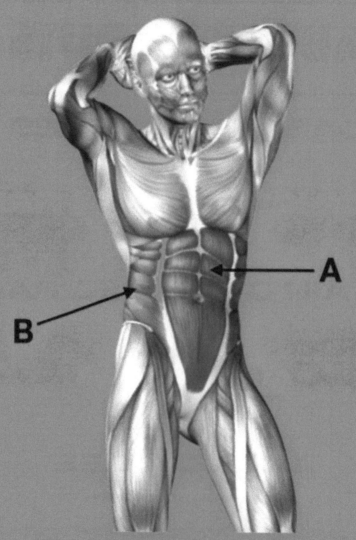

A = RECTUS ABDOMINIS (6-Pack)
B = EXTERNAL ABDOMINAL OBLIQUES

(INVISIBLE ABDOMINAL MUSCLES)

(Lying behind the outer visible muscles)

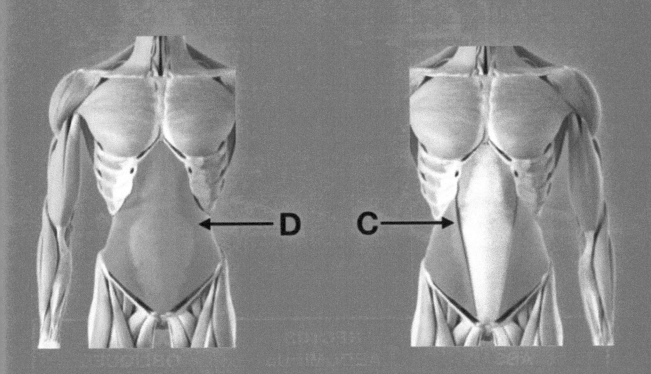

C = INTERNAL ABDOMINAL OBLIQUES

D= TRANSVERSUS ABDOMINIS

ABDOMINAL WORKOUTS

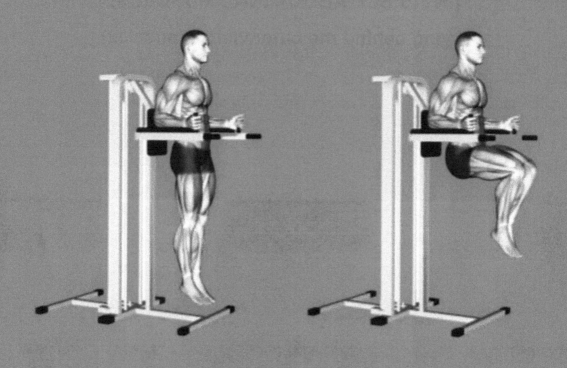

ENTIRE ABS	RECTUS ABDOMINUS	EXTERNAL OBLIQUES
Hanging Leg Raises	Captain Chair Leg Raises	Captain Chair Leg Raises
Cable Crunches	Cable Crunches	Cable Crunches
Air Bicycles	Ab Roller	
Decline Abdominal Crunches		

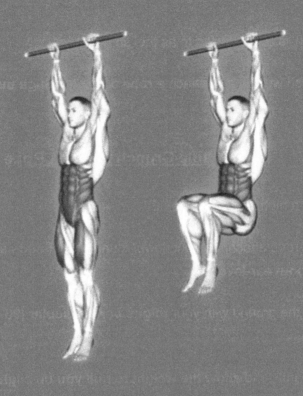

INTERNAL OBLIQUES	TRANSVERSE ABDOMINALS
Captain Chair Leg Raises	Air Bicycles
Cable Crunches	Bird Dog Crunch
Air Bicycles	Planks
	Ab Roller

CABLE CRUNCHES

- The 'cable-crunch' is also referred to as the 'ab pulldown'

- Select your desired weight, and attach a **rope** or **bar** to a **high pulley**.

Cable Crunch Using A Rope

1. Attach a rope to a high pulley (Figure 53).

2. Grasp the cable rope attachment and lower it until **your hands are placed next to your face (about ear-level).**

3. **Kneel down** on the ground with your **thighs perpendicular (90 degrees) to the ground.**

4. Flex your hips slightly and **allow the weight to pull you up slightly until you hyperextend and arch your lower back.** This will be your **starting position.**

5. From the starting position, **pull your elbows down to the middle of your thighs/knees** whilst contracting your abs and **folding your torso inwards.** Exhale whilst doing this movement. Once your elbows touch your mid-thigh/knee region, that will be your **finishing position.**

6. Hold in this position for one second before **slowly** returning back to **the starting position.**

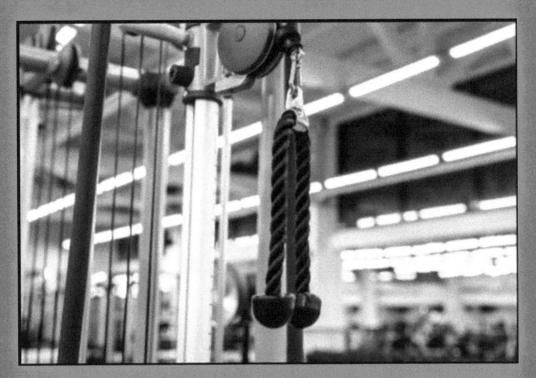

Figure 53: *Rope* attached to a high pulley.

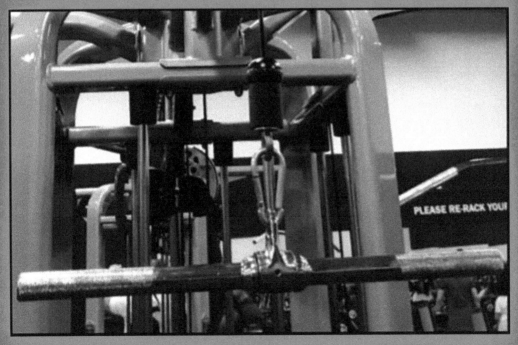

Figure 54: *Bar* attached to a high pulley.

Cable Crunch Using A Bar

1. **Grab the bar** (Figure 54) **on the inside** so that the **palms are facing your body**.

2. Bring the bar down as you kneel down.

3. Hold bar **behind your neck** whilst **keeping your head up** (i.e., bar is in contact with back of the neck).

4. **Kneel down** on the ground with your **thighs perpendicular (90 degrees) to the ground**.

5. Flex your hips slightly and **allow the weight to pull you up slightly until you hyperextend the lower back**. This will be your **starting position**.

6. From the starting position, **pull your elbows down to your knees/middle of the thighs** whilst contracting your abs and **folding your torso inwards**. Exhale whilst doing this movement.

7. Once your elbows touch your mid-thigh/knee region, that will be your **finishing position**.

8. Hold in this position for one second before **slowly** returning back to **the starting position**.

Useful Tips

- Make sure that you keep **constant tension on the abs throughout the movement**.

- **Do not** keep your back arched throughout the entire movement. **Your back should only be arched when you're returning back to starting position**.

- Make sure the weight is **not too heavy** otherwise your back will take the brunt of the work as opposed to your abs.

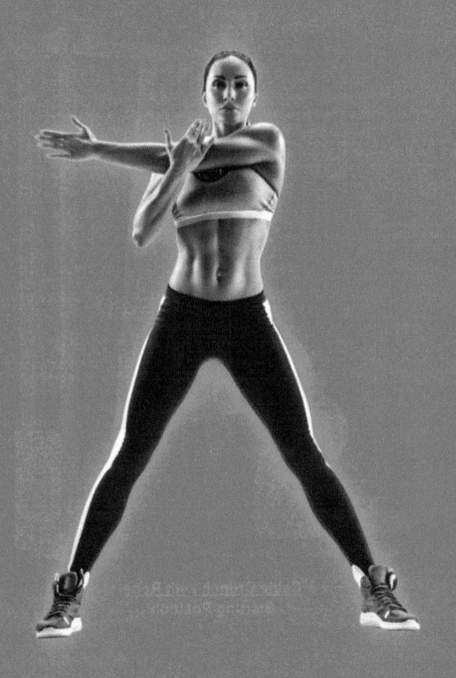

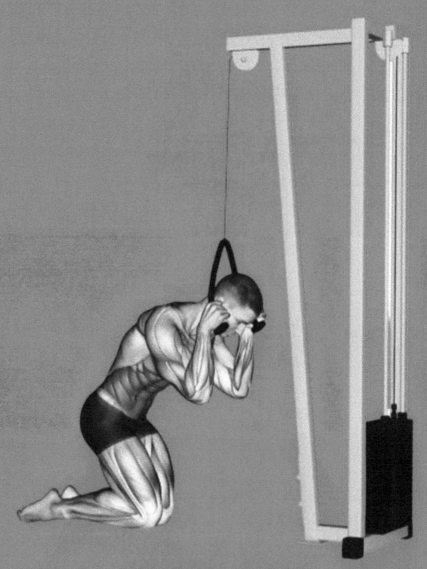

Cable Crunch with Rope
Starting Position

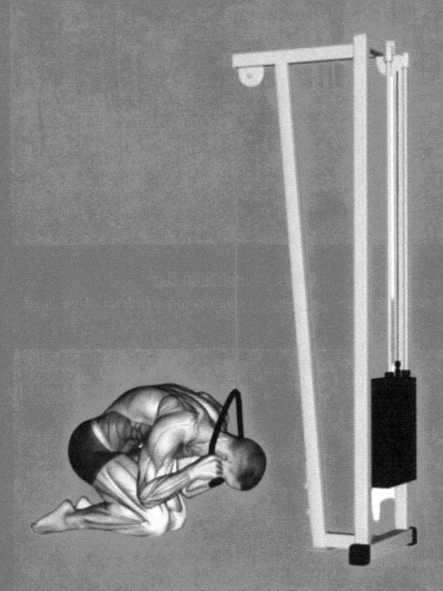

<u>Cable Crunch with Rope</u>
Finishing Position

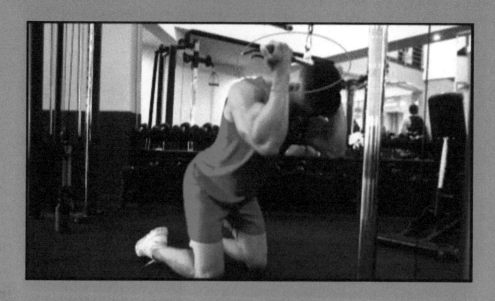

Cable Crunch with Bar

Grab Bar from the Inside and Ensure Contact with Back of the Head.

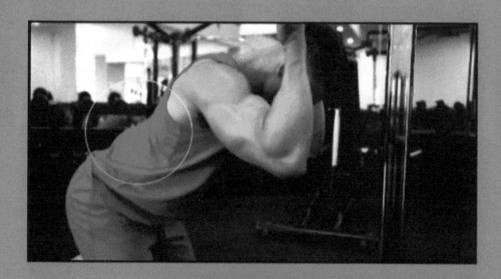

Cable Crunch with Bar

Start position with Hyperextended/ Arched Lower Back.

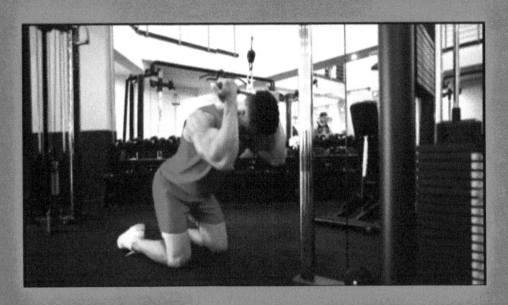

Cable Crunch with Bar
Starting Position

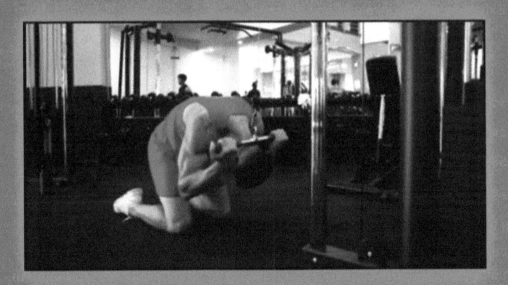

Cable Crunch with Bar
Finishing Position

HANGING LEG RAISES

- Use the **'pull-up bar'** (Figure 55) for this exercise.

1. Grab bar at a slightly **wider than shoulder-width** with an **overhand grip** so that **palms are facing the floor**.

2. Bring your feet together and straight.

3. Keep your core tight.

4. Lift your knees as high as you can **whilst they're together**.

5. **Keep your legs in front of your body** at all times.

6. Hold for a second before returning to starting position.

7. Exhale as you lift, inhale as you descend.

Useful Tips

- Some trainees experience a lot of stress on their shoulders when doing this exercise. It's not a bad idea, therefore, to purchase some **'ab straps'** (Figure 56)and attach them to the pull-up bar to **alleviate this unwanted stress** and get your abs to do all the work.

- **If you find yourself swinging forwards and backwards** a lot in the beginning, just start off hanging of the bar and engaging your core. **Focus on using your core to keep yourself still**, and **keep your feet straight and firm**. With time, you will get used to it and become stable.

- You want to **lift your straight legs/knees as high as you can** so as to engage the abs more (especially the lower abs).

- Keep your tension in the ab region at all times. Maintain a smooth and controlled movement throughout **so as to minimise any swinging**.

- **An alternative to the knee raise is the leg raise**. Here, the legs are kept straight and at a 90 degree angle to the torso.

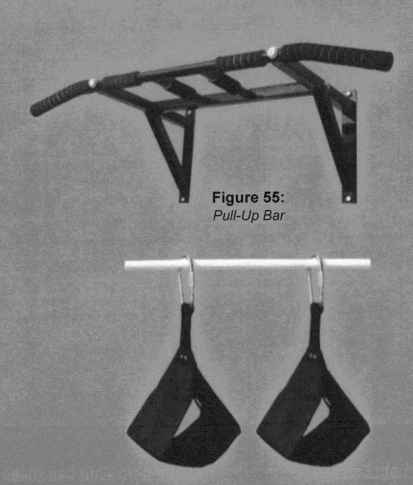

Figure 55:
Pull-Up Bar

Figure 56:
Ab Straps

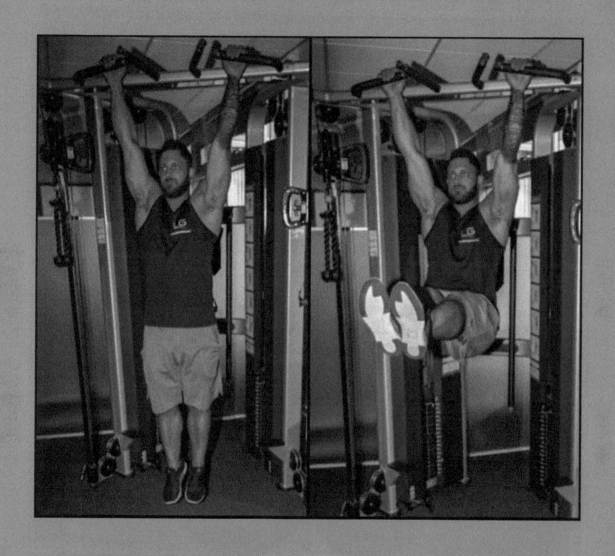

Hanging Straight Leg Raise

Starting Position

Hanging Straight Leg Raise

Finishing Position

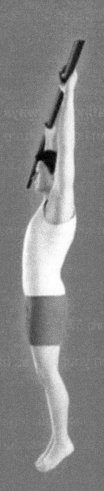

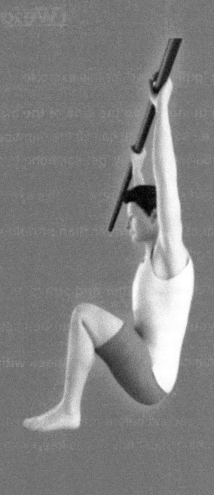

Hanging Knee Raise

Starting Position

Hanging Knee Raise

Finishing Position

HANGING KNEE/LEG RAISES
(Weighted)

- Use the **'pull-up bar'** for this exercise.

- **Place a dumbbell on the side of the machine** so that it's **resting sideways on its plate** (i.e., so that you can lift the dumbbell with your feet when hanging from the pull-up bar). Alternately, get someone to put it in place for you.

- Ideally, use some 'ab straps' for this exercise routine.

1. Grab bar at **slightly wider than shoulder-width** with an overhand grip so that palms are facing the floor.

2. Bring your **feet together and straight**.

3. **Using your feet, grab the dumbbell** between your feet (Figure 57).

4. Keep your core tight. Lift your **knees with the weight** between your feet as high as you can.

5. Hold for a second before returning to starting position. Do **not** allow your legs to swing behind your body. Try to keep your **legs in front of you** at all times during the routine.

6. Exhale as you lift, inhale as you descend.

Useful Tips

- Start off with a light weight and get used to this exercise before progressing to heavier weights. Starting off too heavy can lead to excessive rocking forwards and backwards, as well as increase the chance of a potential back injury.

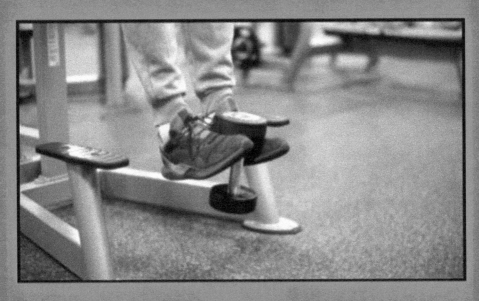

Figure 57:

Using Your Feet, Grab the Dumbbell Once Set Up for the 'Weighted Knee/Leg Raise.'

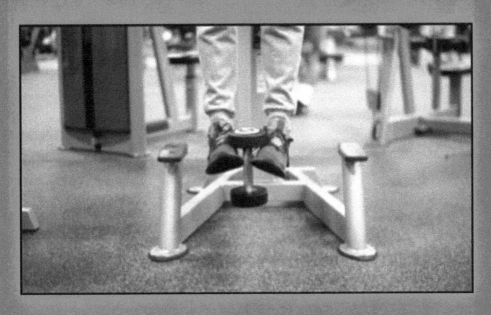

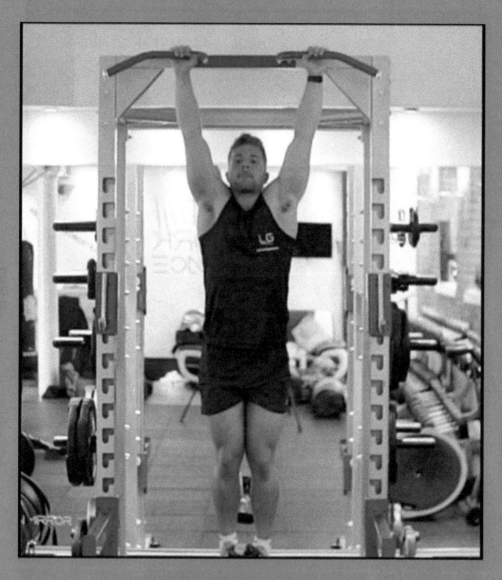

Weighted <u>Hanging Knee Raise</u>

Starting Position

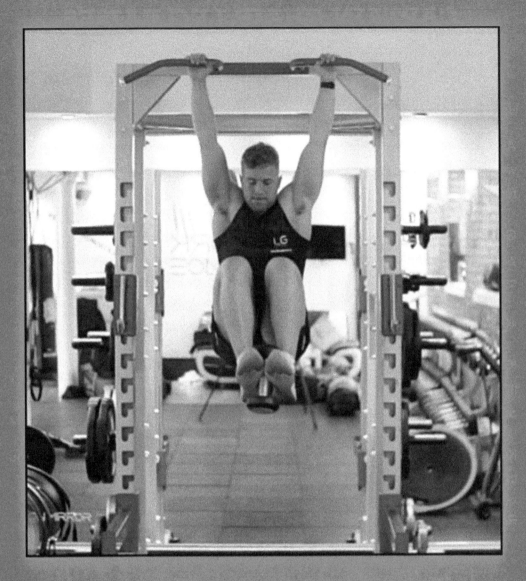

Weighted <u>Hanging Knee Raise</u>

Finishing Position

CAPTAIN CHAIR LEG RAISES

VERSION ONE - KNEE RAISE

- Use the 'pull-up bar' for this exercise.

- As with the 'weighted hanging leg raise,' this exercise can be done weighted. Just pick up the dumbbell (that's lying on its side) with your feet.

1. Get into position on the **'captain chair leg raise'** machine by putting your **arms on the arm pads** and hold onto the handles as tight as you can.

2. Make sure your back is **snug firmly against the back pad**.

3. Keep your **feet together**, straight and hanging off the ground. However, they should be **slightly in front of your body**. This is your **starting position**.

4. Keep your torso tight, take a deep breath and **lift your knees up as high as you can**. Hold for a second before returning to your starting position.

5. Repeat.

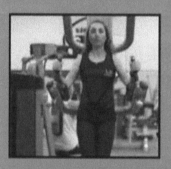
Captain Chair Knee Raise
Starting Position

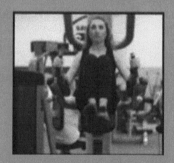
Captain Chair Knee Raise
Finishing Position

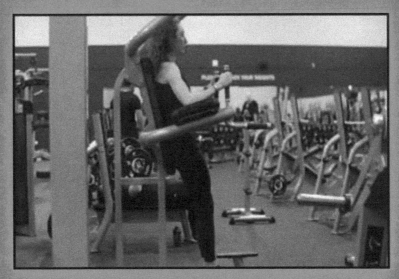

Captain Chair Knee Raise
Starting Position

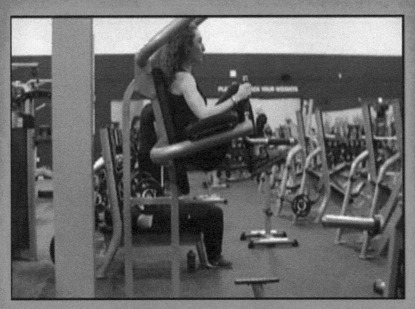

Captain Chair Knee Raise
Finishing Position

- Use the 'pull-up bar' for this exercise.

- As with the 'weighted hanging leg raise,' this exercise can be done weighted. Just pick up the dumbbell (that's lying on its side) with your feet.

1. Get into position on the **'captain chair leg raise'** machine by putting your arms on the arm pads and hold onto the handles as tight as you can.

2. Make sure your back is snug firmly against the back pad.

3. **Keep your feet together, straight and hanging off the ground**. However, they should be slightly in front of your body with your toes facing upwards. This is your starting position.

4. Keep your torso tight, take a deep breath and, whilst **keeping your legs straight, rotate your legs upwards and forwards as high as you can**.

5. Hold for a second before returning to your starting position.

6. Repeat.

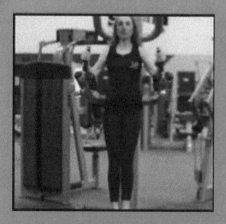

Captain Chair Straight Leg Raise
Starting Position

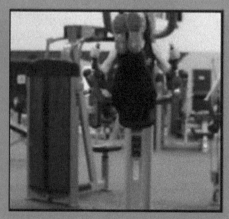

Captain Chair Straight Leg Raise
Starting Position

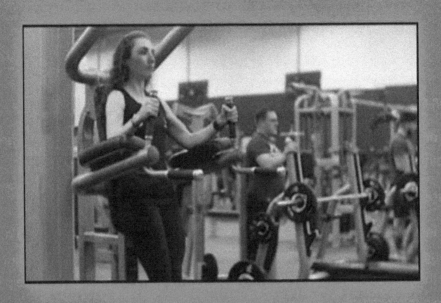

Captain Chair Straight Leg Raise
Starting Position

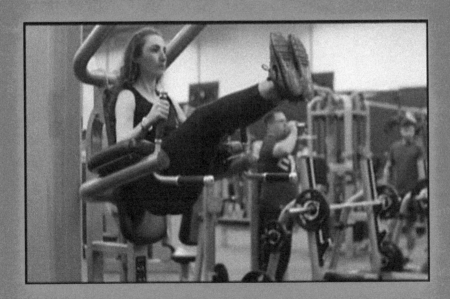

Captain Chair Straight Leg Raise
Finishing Position

AB ROLLER

1. Get an **ab roller** (Figure 58) or **barbell** (Figure 59).

2. **Start on the your hands and knees**. Make sure that the floor is smooth and unobstructed.

3. Hold the bars on either side of the wheel or barbell at shoulder-width.

4. **Suck in your abs** and put yourself into a position as if you're about to do a kneeling push up. In other words, **keep your arms straight onto the roller** whilst the roller is in front of your head. **Keeping your head down** will help you maintain this posture.

5. Take a deep breath then **slowly roll the ab-roller** forwards maintaining a tight torso.

6. Continue until your **body is straight**. Stop **just before your body touches the floor**.

7. Pause for 2-3 seconds at this position and then return to starting position as you exhale.

Useful Tips

- The trick is to **go slowly at all times** whilst maintaining a tight core.

- You can use this exercise to **train your obliques** by moving the ab roller diagonally instead of straight.

- Don't let your bottom sag toward the ground at any point. Imagine there's a **long, flat plank** on your back, from your head to your tailbone.

- When you become more skilled and are ready to 'up the intensity,' you can perform this exercise from a 'standing-up' position as opposed to on your knees

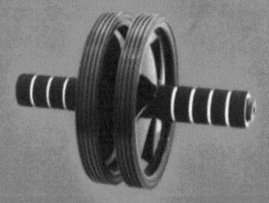

Figure 58:

Ab Roller

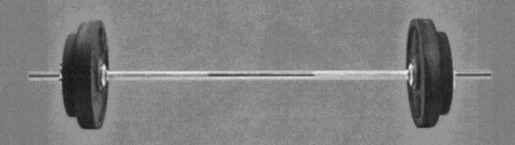

Figure 59:

Barbell

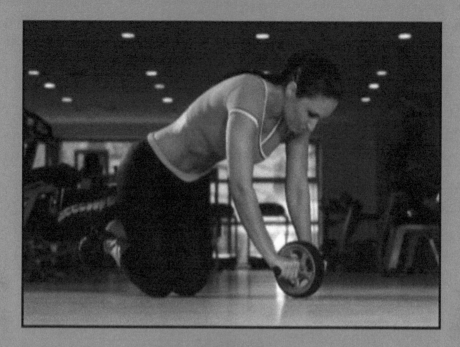

Ab Roller Exercise (with 'Ab Roller')
Starting Position

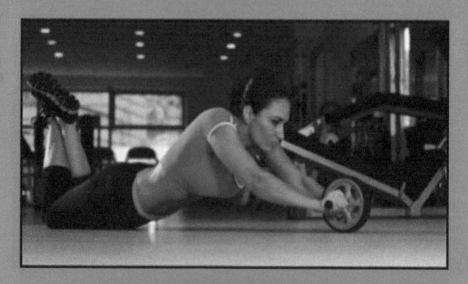

Ab Roller Exercise (with 'Ab Roller')
Finishing Position

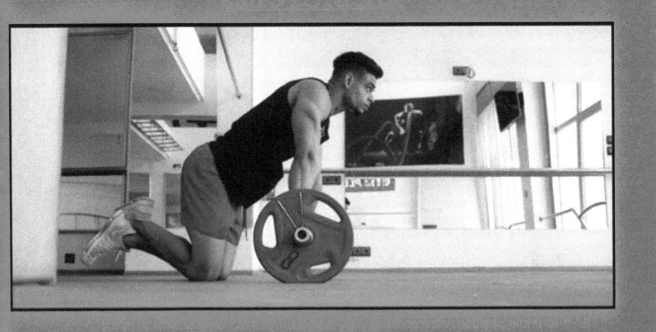

<u>Ab Roller Exercise (with Barbell)</u>
Starting Position

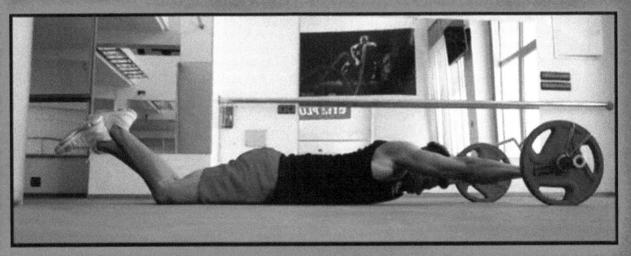

<u>Ab Roller Exercise (with Barbell)</u>
Finishing Position

265

AIR BICYCLES

1. Lie flat on the ground with your **lower back pressed firmly against the ground**.

2. **Bend your knees** and rest your feet flat against the floor.

3. Lift your head into the **crunch position** and **place your hands next to your head** (Figure 60). Be careful not to strain your neck as you perform it.

4. **Raise your knees up until they are perpendicular (90 degrees) to the floor**, with your **lower legs (calves) parallel to the floor**. This will be your starting position.

5. From this position, start moving your legs as if you're riding a bicycle in the air. In other words, slowly go through a cycle pedal motion by **kicking forward with the left leg and bringing in the knee of the right leg**.

6. At the same time, **bring your left elbow close to your right knee** by crunching to the side, as you breathe out (Figure 61)

7. Repeat this alternating the motion to failure.

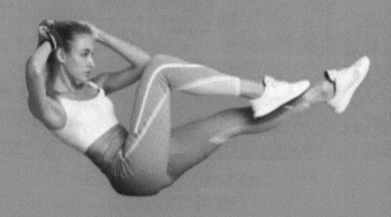

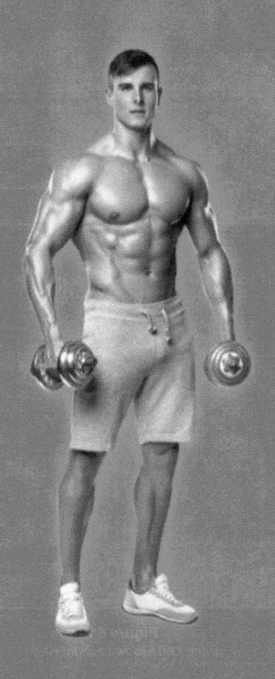

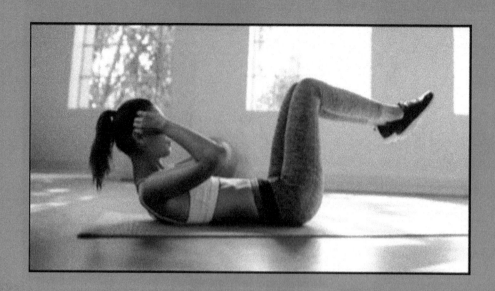

Figure 60:
Lift Your Head into Crunch Position and Place Your Hands Next to Your Head.

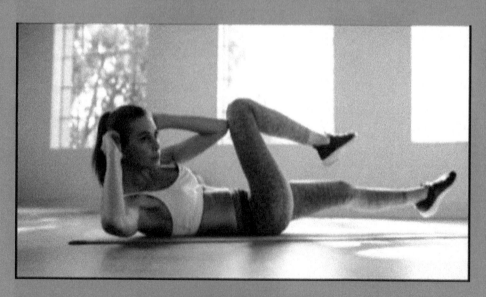

Figure 61:
Bring Left Elbow to Right Knee.

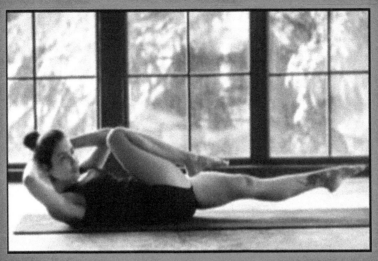

<u>Air Bicycles Exercise</u>
(Left Elbow to Right Knee)

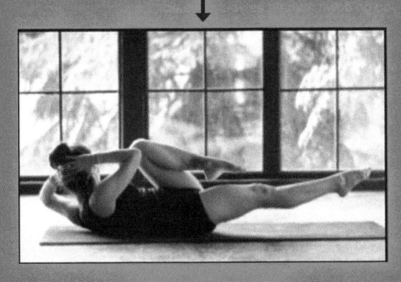

<u>Air Bicycles Exercise</u>
(Right Elbow to Left Knee)

DECLINE CRUNCH

1. Find an adjustable **'sit-up' bench** and adjust to the **decline position** (Figure 62). The more declined the bench is, the more difficult the exercise.

2. **Secure your legs** at the end of the bench and lie down.

3. Arch your back slightly and maintain this position.

4. **Cross your arms in front of your chest** as you sit up and keep your core tight at all times.

5. You can choose to **come up all the way, or you can come up half way**. Coming up half way before returning to starting position will keep the intensity in your abs making the exercise much harder.

6. Inhale as you go down, exhale as you come up.

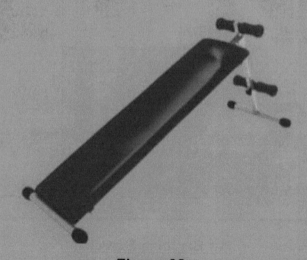

Figure 62:

Decline 'Sit-Up' Bench.

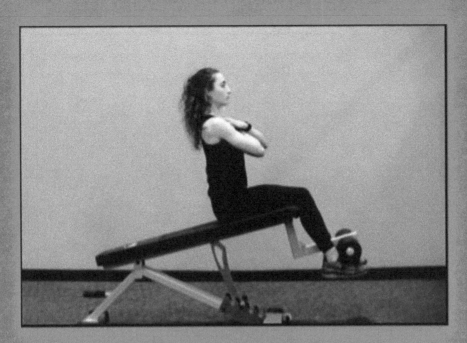

Decline Crunch
(Starting Position)

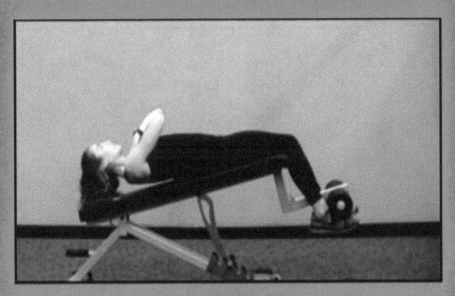

Decline Crunch
(Finishing Position)

271

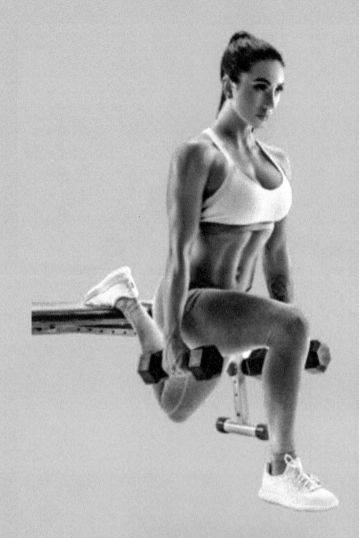

BUTT
WORKOUTS

BUTT WORKOUTS

DEADLIFT

SQUATS

HIP THRUSTS

ROMANIAN DEADLIFTS

BULGARIAN SPLIT SQUATS

DONKEY KICKS

MUSCLES OF THE BUTT

(GLUTEAL MUSCLES)

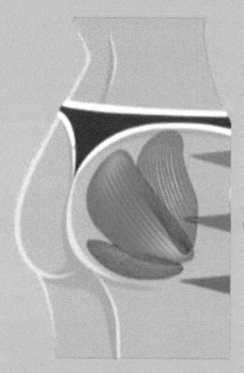

GLUTEUS MEDIUS

GLUTEUS MAXIMUS

GLUTEUS MINIMUS

GLUTEUS MAXIMUS
GLUTEUS MEDIUS
GLUTEUS MINIMUS

BUTT WORKOUTS

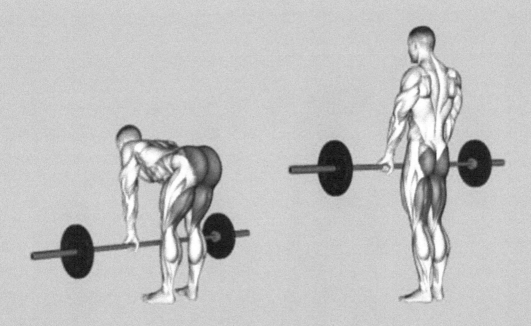

ENTIRE BUTT	GLUTEUS MAXIMUS	GLUTEUS MEDIUS	GLUTEUS MINIMUS
Squats (Deep)	Deadlift	Deadlift	Sideplank
Hip Thrust	Romanian Deadlift	Burpees	Bulgarian Split Squats
Bulgarian Split Squats	Butt-Blaster (Donkey-Kick)		

BUTT WORKOUTS:
An Overview

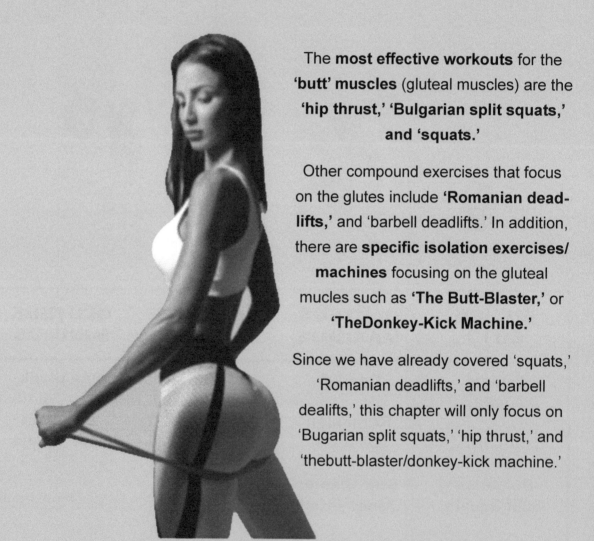

The **most effective workouts** for the 'butt' muscles (gluteal muscles) are the **'hip thrust,' 'Bulgarian split squats,' and 'squats.'**

Other compound exercises that focus on the glutes include **'Romanian dead-lifts,'** and 'barbell deadlifts.' In addition, there are **specific isolation exercises/ machines** focusing on the gluteal mucles such as **'The Butt-Blaster,'** or **'TheDonkey-Kick Machine.'**

Since we have already covered 'squats,' 'Romanian deadlifts,' and 'barbell dealifts,' this chapter will only focus on 'Bugarian split squats,' 'hip thrust,' and 'thebutt-blaster/donkey-kick machine.'

HIP THRUSTS

1. Grab a bench and **put your shoulders against the side of it**. Ideally ensure the bench is stable and difficult to topple over.

2. **Spread your arms across the top of the bench for stability** (If your shoulders don't reach the bench, you may need to start with your butt slightly off the floor).

3. **Bend your knees to a 90 degree angle** whilst keeping your **feet flat on the floor and shoulder-width apart**.

4. Ideally, do this exercise in front of a mirror. Keep your head facing the mirror and **keep looking straight throughout the exercise** (Doing this helps to protect your spine).

5. Tighten your core and take a deep breath.

6. As you exhale, **squeeze your glutes as you lift your hips upwards**.

7. At the top position, **your torso and thighs should be parallel to the floor**.

8. When you reach the top position, you want to make sure you're **squeezing your glutes as hard as you can for a second or so.**

9. Slowly return to the starting position.

Additional Tips

- Do not use any weight at all **until you've mastered the form first**.

- You can use a **barbell** or weight to add more difficulty to the exercise.

- If you're using the barbell to do this exercise, then **place the bar on your hips and use your hands to keep bar stable** (Figure 63).

- Proceed with caution if you've had a lower back injury.

- Do not hyperextend your spine. In the top position, as you're looking forward, the torso and thighs should look relatively flat. **There's no need to go any higher**.

- Make sure your **feet remain flat on the floor**.

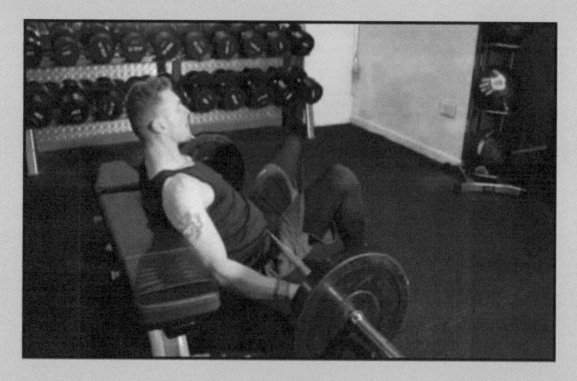

Figure 63:

Place the Bar on Your Hips.

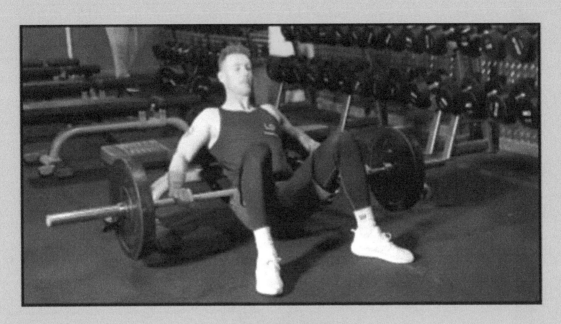

Hip Thrust
Starting Position

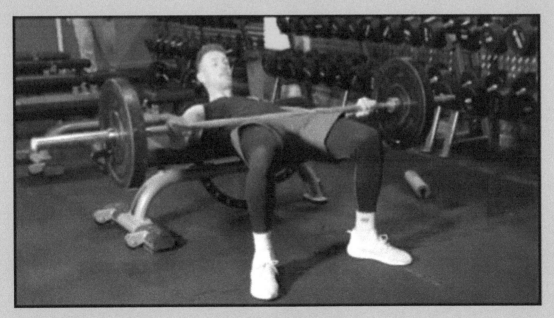

Hip Thrust
Finishing Position

279

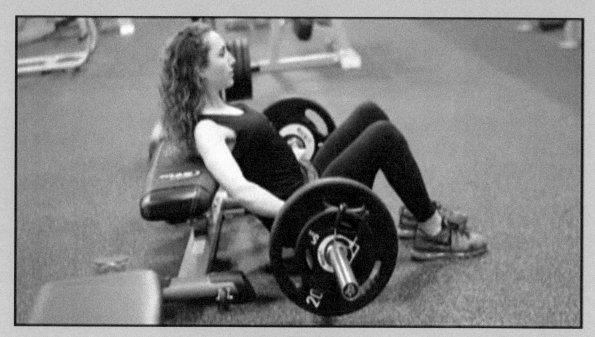

<u>Hip Thrust</u>
Starting Position

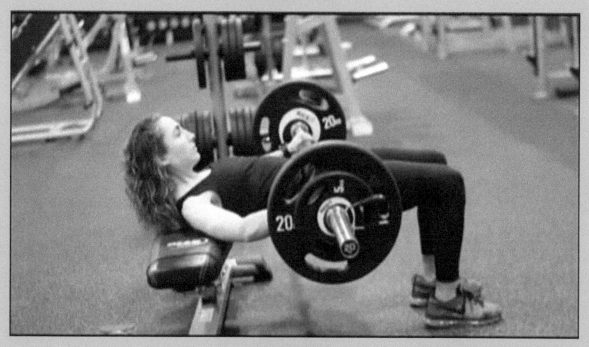

<u>Hip Thrust</u>
Finishing Position
280

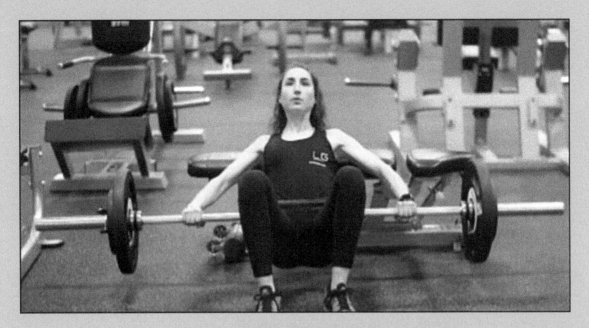

Hip Thrust
Starting Position

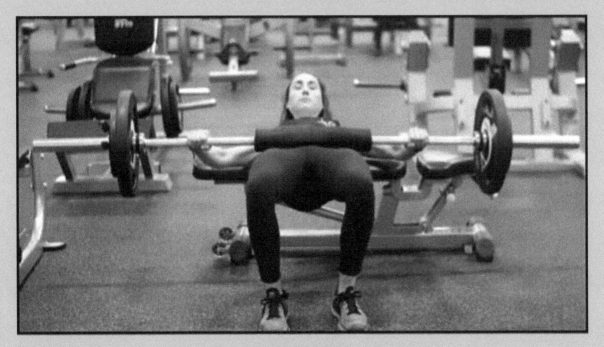

Hip Thrust
Starting Position

BULGARIAN SPLIT SQUATS

1. Grab a bench, and **place your right foot (front foot) standing in a forward position** whilst your **left leg is on a bench**.

2. Your **front leg** is going to be the **'working' leg** in this exercise whereas the 'back' leg will be utilised for balance.

3. You can either have the **rear foot flat on the bench** (i.e. laces on your trainers touching bench surface) or on **your toes** (heels in the air).

4. Inhale, keep your **core tight and chest up** as you go into a deep lunge until the **knee of the back foot is almost touching the floor**. At the same time, **ensure the knee of the front leg does not shoot in front of your toes**. If it does, then create more space between your feet by moving your front leg forwards.

5. Exhale and push through the **heel of your front foot** as you return back to the starting position.

6. Once you've done your designated number of reps, swap over and **do the same with the other (left) leg**.

Bodyweight Alone

- If you're using **bodyweight alone**, then keep your hands together with fingers inter locked in a **prayer position**. Alternatively, you can keep your **hands by your side** or in front of you to help keep balance during the movement.

Barbell in Squat Position

• **A very popular variation** of this exercise involves using a barbell placed on your traps (as if you're doing a squat) as opposed to dumbbells.

Dumbbell Weights in Each Hand

• When you're ready to use weights, you can do this exercise **using a dumbbell in each hand**. Ensure a tight core and keep your **back and chest upright** whilst doing so.

Additional Tips

• As an option, you can place a pad/towel on the ground in the position where the back knee goes to on its descent. This can provide you with a **reliable** indication with regards to how low down to go. It also helps **protect your knee** from accidentally hitting the floor.

• The majority of your weight should be **shifted towards your front leg**.

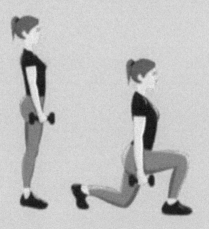

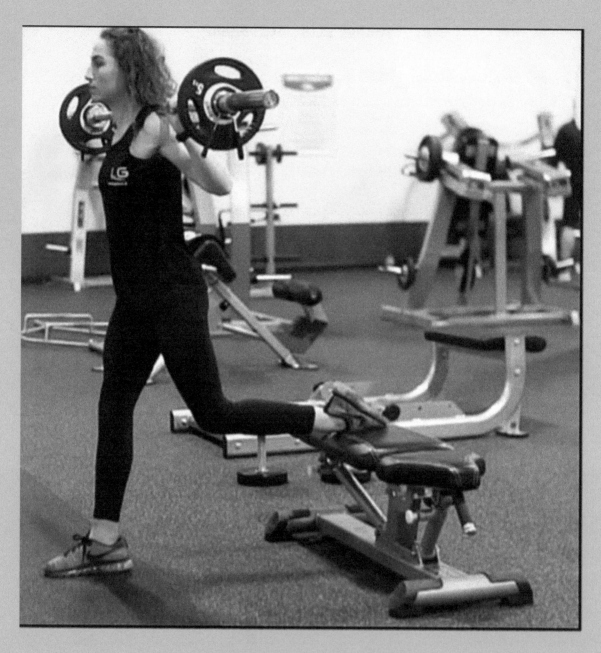

<u>Bulgarian Split Squat (with Barbell)</u>

Starting Position

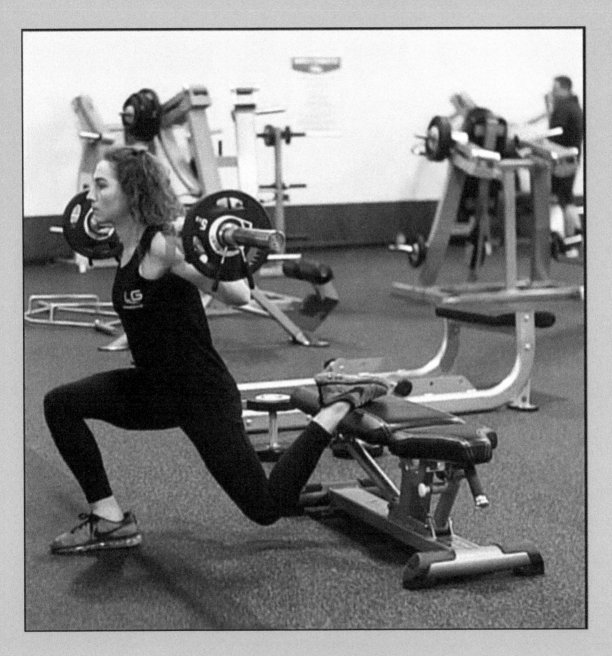

Bulgarian Split Squat (with Barbell)

Finishing Position

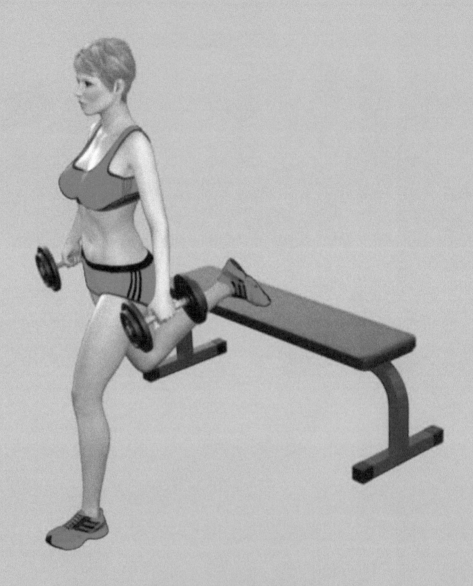

<u>Bulgarian Split Squat (with Dumbbells)</u>

Starting Position

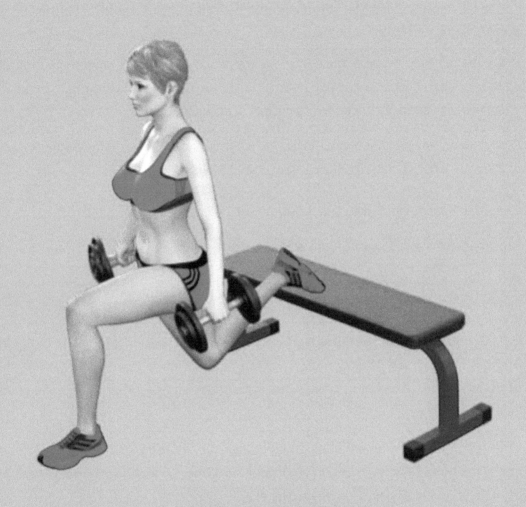

<u>Bulgarian Split Squat (with Dumbbells)</u>

Finishing Position

DONKEY-KICK/BUTT BLASTER

- Most gyms will have a **'butt blaster' machine, 'glute-master,' 'donkey-kick' machine** or something similar to it.

- These machines/isolation exercises alone are not as effective as hip thrusts, deadlifts or squats for gluteal muscle development, but they are **excellent adjuncts** to these exercises and certainly have a place in your gym routine.

- The following advice should be applicable in either case, but if you're unsure (as with all of these exercises), then please contact a staff member in the gym.

1. Enter the machine and **grab the handles in front**.

2. Ensure the **abs are drawn in and torso is tight**.

3. Position your feet so that there's a 90 degree angle between your thighs and your torso.

4. Put the **right foot (the 'working leg') on the rear 'foot' pad** of the machine (Figure 64). **Stand on the left leg (the 'non-working leg') and place it against the pad at the front of the machine**. (on most machines, the front pad would rest against your shins and take a deep breath.

5. Breathe out as you extend the right leg **backwards as far as you can** whilst keeping the rest of the body stationary. Ensure your **hips and body are straight and parallel** to the centre (i.e., avoid any rotation of your hips).

6. Focus on **contracting the glutes** when you reach the top position.

7. Hold for a second before returning to your starting position.

8. Carry out your designated number of reps before **switching over to the other leg**.

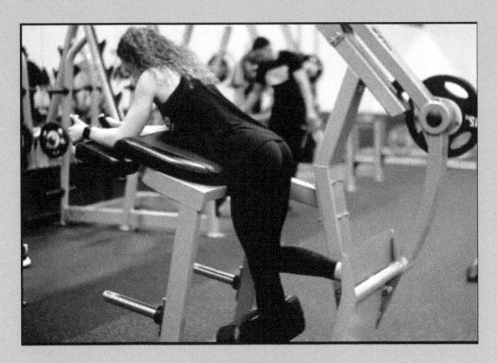

'Donkey-Kick' Machine
Starting Position

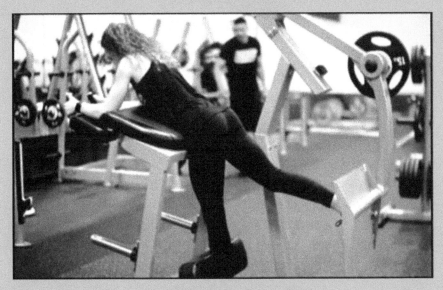

'Donkey-Kick' Machine
Finishing Position

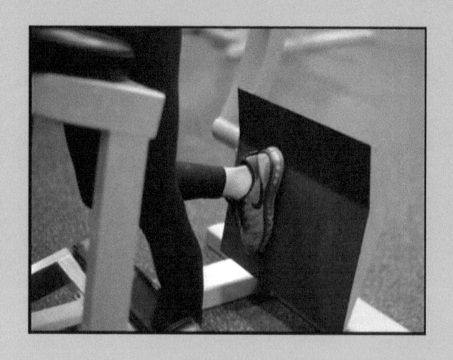

Figure 64:

Place right foot agains pad whilst left leg is against the shin pad.

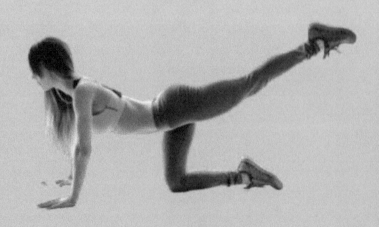

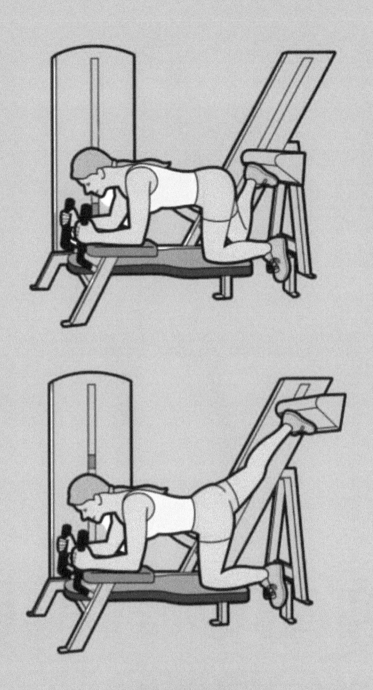

'Donkey-Kick'/
Butt-Blaster Machine

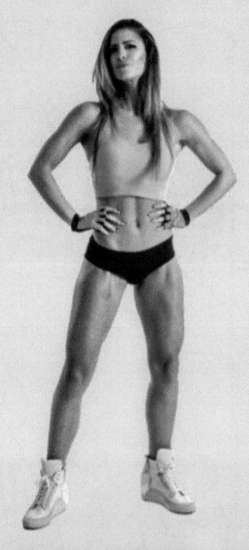

ROTATORY CUFF
WORKOUTS

ROTATORY CUFF WORKOUTS

FACEPULL

DUMBBELL INTERNAL ROTATION

DUMBBELL EXTERNAL ROTATION

ROTATORY CUFF MUSCLES

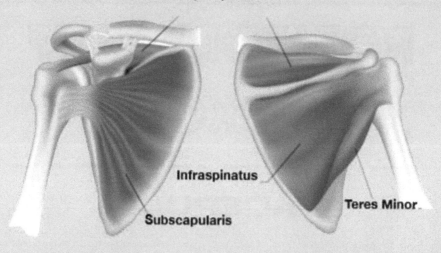

Supraspinatus

Infraspinatus

Subscapularis

Teres Minor

ANTERIOR VIEW

POSTERIOR VIEW

The rotator cuff muscles provide
strength and stability to the
shoulder, especially during
movement.

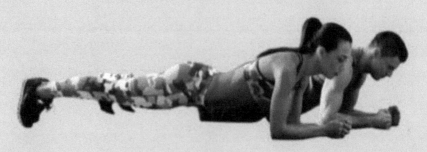

ROTATORY CUFF WORKOUTS

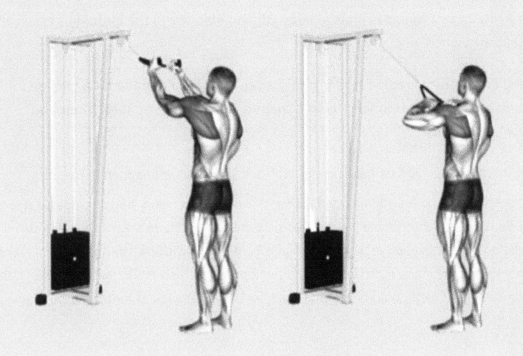

ROTATORY CUFF MUSCLES
Facepull
Dumbbell Internal Rotation
Dumbbell External Rotation

ROTATORY CUFF EXERCISES

- **The rotator cuff muscles** provide **strength and stability to the shoulder**, especially during movement (Figure 65).

- Tendons at the ends of the rotator cuff muscles are **prone to becoming torn or damaged though prolonged weight training sessions or general 'wear and tear'** (Figure 66).

- Inflammation/damage to these rotator cuff muscles is not uncommon in trainees undergoing exercises such as military press, shoulder press or bench press on a regular basis. The risk, unfortunately, is further increased when these exercises are done with poor posture or excessively heavy weights. **To prevent/reduce chance of injury**, we should not only make sure we're doing the aforementioned prescribed exercise routines with **excellent form**, but **also** perform 'rotator cuff' exercises **at least once a week.**

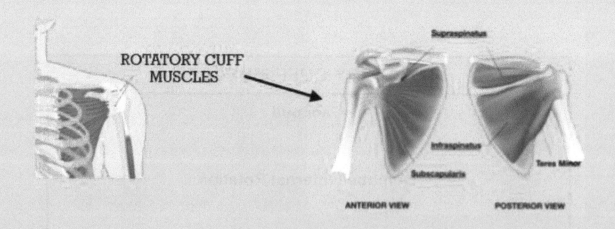

Figure 65:

*Rotatory Cuff Muscles provide
Strength and Stability to the Shoulder.*

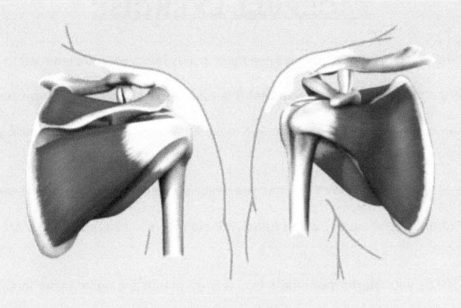

Figure 66:

Tendons at the Ends of the Rotator Cuff Muscles can be Prone to Inflammation and 'wear & tear.'

NORMAL   ROTATORY CUFF PROBLEMS

Inflamed/torn tendons

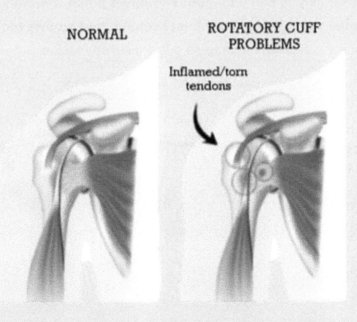

FACEPULL EXERCISE

1. The best equipment for a face pull is a cable pulley machine. Attach a rope to the pulley.

2. Position the **top of the pulley so that it is just above the height of your head**.

3. Take an **overhand grip** of the rope and make sure your **thumbs are pointing towards the back of the room**.

4. Take a few steps back from the machine whilst **shoulders are dropped/lower position**.

5. **Feet should be shoulder width apart**. For stability, you can put one foot forward and one back.

6. This will be your **starting position**; take a deep breath and tighten your torso.

7. Pull the **rope towards your face (eye-level)** ensuring that the **elbows are higher than your wrist** at all times. Always make sure you are **leaning slightly backward rather than forward**.

8. Go back **as far as you can until your shoulders pinch**. You want to focus on **squeezing the shoulder blades whilst keeping your elbows higher than your wrists**. Return to starting position remembering to exhale on release.

"So, when I'm referring to the 'Facepull' exercise, I don't mean this."

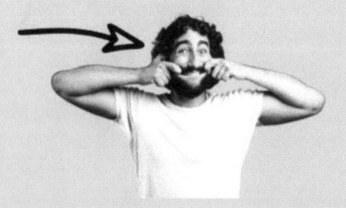

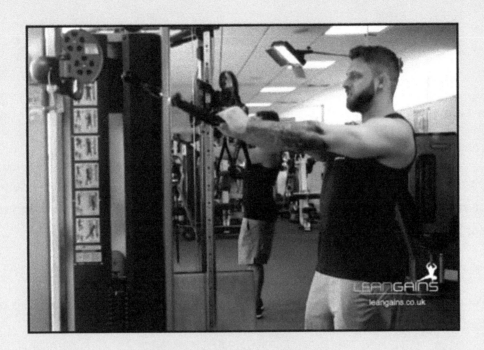

<u>Facepull</u> - Starting Position

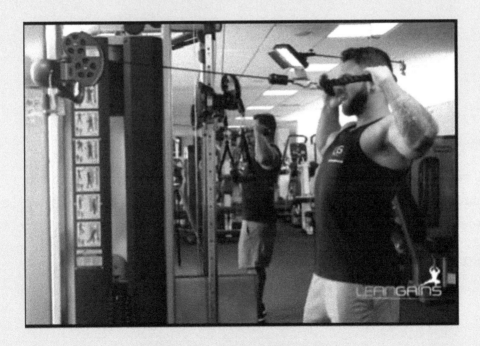

<u>Facepull</u> - Finishing Position

DUMBBELL INTERNAL ROTATION

1. **Lie sideways on an exercise bench** (or on the floor) resting on your upper back.

2. Grab a dumbbell with an **underside grip** (palm facing upwards).

3. **Keep your elbow in contact with the bench** (or floor) and extend your **forearm outwards so that it's angled at 90 degrees to your biceps and parallel to the floor**.

4. This will be your **starting position**.

5. Take a deep breath and exhale as you raise and rotate the dumbbell from the bench/ floor towards the centre.

6. Hold for a second before returning to the starting position.

7. Repeat.

Additional Tips

- Keep your **upper arm in tight contact with your body** during the whole movement.

- Maintain a **smooth momentum** throughout the exercise.

- You **cannot** perform internal rotation with a dumbbell while standing upright, because gravity does not provide resistance for the rotator cuff. You have to lie across a flat exercise bench or on the floor.

- **Keep the weight light**. There's no need to go heavy with these exercises.

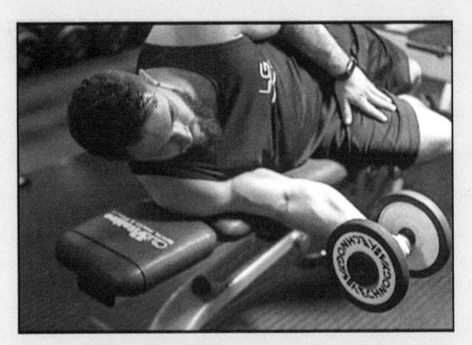

<u>Dumbbell Internal Rotation</u>- Starting Position

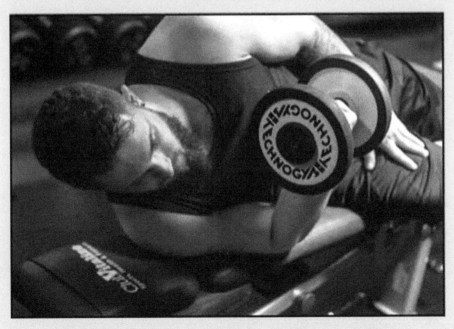

<u>Dumbbell Internal Rotation</u>- Finishing Position

301

DUMBBELL EXTERNAL ROTATION

1. **Lie sideways on a bench** so that your **left arm** is resting on the floor or holding the bench for support.

2. **Grab a dumbbell with your right hand** and an overhand (palms down) grip.

3. Bend the elbow so that it's **90-degrees between the upper arm and the forearm**.

4. In other words, the **forearm should be parallel to the floor whilst perpendicular to your torso**. The **upper arm** should be stationary next to your torso and **also parallel to the floor.**

5. **Rotate the dumbbell in an upward arc away from the floor towards the ceiling** whilst keeping the upper arm and elbow **in contact with the body. Only the forearm should be moving**.

6. Return to **starting position** and repeat. Remember to exhale on the ascend and inhale on the descend.

Additional Tips

- Keep your upper arm in tight contact with your body during the whole movement.
- Maintain a smooth momentum throughout the exercise.
- **Keep the weight light**. There's no need to go heavy with these exercises.

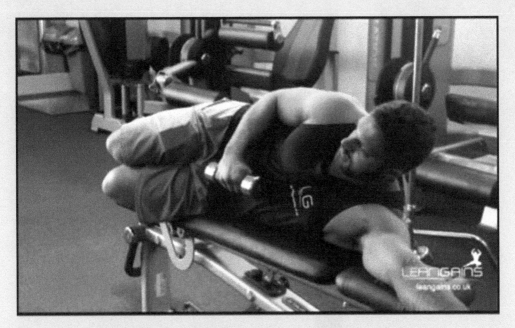

Dumbbell External Rotation - Starting Position

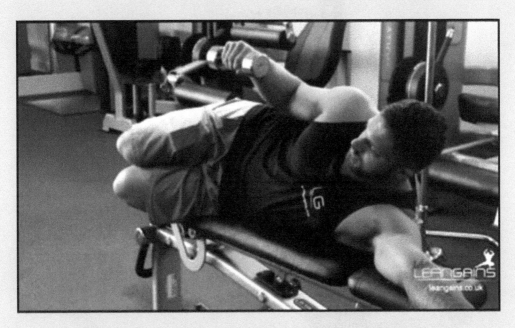

Dumbbell External Rotation - Finishing Position

A FEW WORDS
ABOUT STRETCHING

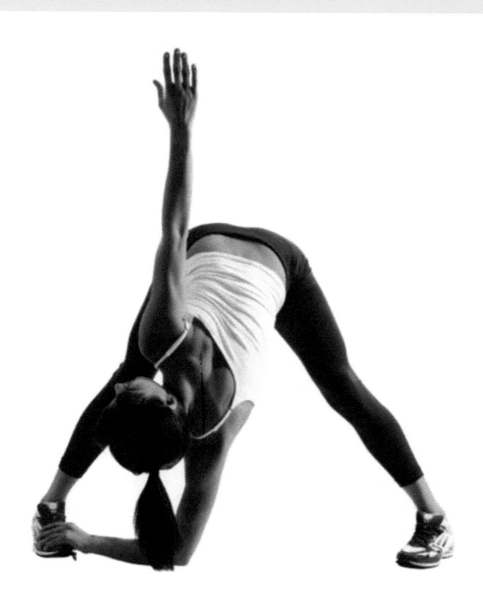

THE BENEFITS OF STRETCHING

Stretching increases flexibility, reduces physical and emotional stress, and increases your range of motion.

In addition, regular stretching increases blood flow and circulation to your muscles which, in turn, reduces recovery time and muscle soreness.

Poor posture is often associated with muscle imbalances. Strength training makes a massive difference in this regard, but so does stretching.

Not only would stretching reduce musculoskeletal pain and discomfort, but can also improve posture and proper alignment.

The biggest advantage associated with stretching is the increased range of motion.

Stretching your muscles on a regular basis allows your joints a wider range of motion allowing for a much greater freedom of movement.

Stretching should be a relatively gentle routine to counterbalance the direct impact of high-intensity of workouts.

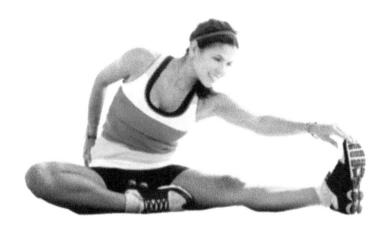

HOW MANY WAYS CAN YOU STRECTH YOUR MUSCLES?

There are many ways you can stretch your muscles, but the main ones are:

Static and Dynamic Stretches

- **Static stretches** involve holding a stretch in a comfortable position for a period of time, typically between 10 and 30 seconds. This form of stretching is most beneficial **after** you exercise.

- **Dynamic stretches** are active movements that cause your muscles to stretch, but the stretch is **not** held in the end position. These stretches are usually done **before** exercise to get your muscles ready for movement.

Dynamic stretches are not as intense as static stretches and can be functional and mimic the movement of the activity or sport you're about to perform. For example, a swimmer may circle their arms before getting into the water. Other examples include lunges with a torso twist.

The light weights indicated prior to your working weight training sets use the same logic here in that they're designed to get your muscles ready for the exercises (or sets in this case).

SHALL I STRETCH BEFORE OR AFTER MY WORKOUT?

A '**cold**' muscle is relatively stiff and stretching it could potentially cause **injury and discomfort**.

306

This is why it's generally advised to stretch after your workout when the muscles are nice and warm.

As a rule of thumb, **stick to the warm-up and pre-workout routine** described in the aforementioned chapters (Option A , Option B, etc.) **as opposed to pre-workout stretching**. Once you've completed your workout, you can **finish off with 5-10 minutes of static stretches**.

On days when you aren't exercising, you should still commit 5-10 minutes of your day to stretching. This would help improve overall flexibility as well as reduce muscle tightness and pain.

<u>A WORD OF ADVICE WHEN IT COMES TO STRETCHING</u>

- **Static stretching** is recommended at the end of your workouts. Breathe deeply while you hold the stretch for **20 to 30 seconds**. Then relax, and repeat the stretch **at least 2 more times**, trying to move a little bit further into it during the second stretch.

- A stretch should NOT be painful. In fact, if stretching is painful, you're going too far. Instead, move into a stretch, and stop when you feel tension.

- If you're feeling pain or discomfort whilst stretching, don't wait for the pain to go away. Instead see a doctor or physiotherapist right away!

- Don't overdo it. If you're stretching the same muscle groups multiple times a day, you risk over-stretching and causing damage.

- Don't bounce! Moving into a stretch and then bouncing is dangerous because it puts way too much pressure on the muscle and associated connective tissue.

STRETCHING AND YOGA

Your cardio routine will improve blood flow throughout the body and help keep your muscles nice and supple.

However, even with cardio, doing these routines on a regular basis may cause your muscles to tighten up after a while causing you to feel less flexible.

This is why it's important to spend **5 minutes** or so stretching after each workout.

It's also a good idea to **start doing yoga**. I would suggest incorporating **at least 2 yoga classes per month** into your routine. Doing this will not only reduce the risk of injury, but also improve your core strength as well as your overall flexibility.

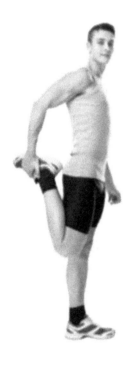
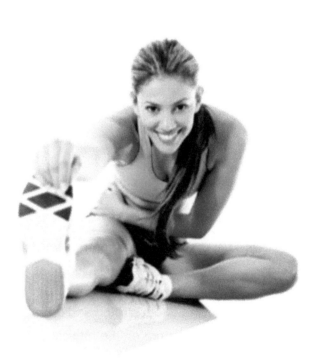

10 ESSENTIAL AFTER WORKOUT STRETCHES

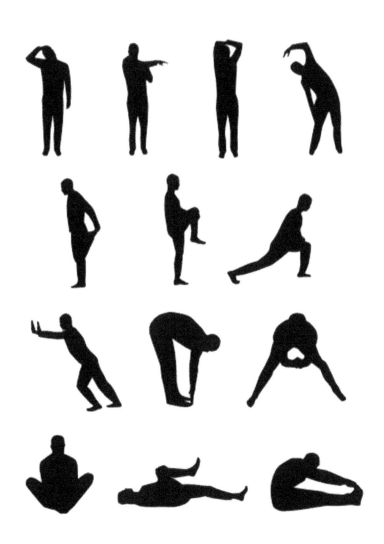

HAMSTRINGS

There are many ways by which you can stretch the hamstring muscles and they are all effective. However, my favourite is the 'standing hamstring stretch.'

The Standing Hamstring Stretch

1. Stand up with straight legs, both feet flat on the floor, and knees straight.

2. Lower your forehead towards your knees whilst bending at the waist until you feel the hamstrings stretch.

3. Hold for 20-30 seconds and repeat twice.

   • If you're very flexible, you can rest your hands on the floor.

   • Alternatively, go down as low as you can **without** over-stretching your hamstrings. Aim to touch your toes.

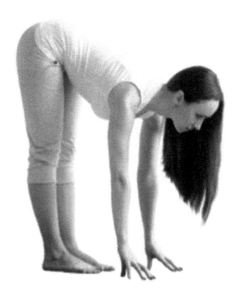

QUADRICEPS

Muscle tension in the **quadriceps** can lead to back and knee pain, overall tightness, and reduced mobility. This is why stretching them is of paramount importance after intense workouts.

Simple Quadricep Stretch

1. Stand upright with feet together.

2. Stand on your left leg whilst grabbing the right leg and pulling it towards your butt. If you're feeling unstable on one leg, you can use a wall or something sturdy to keep yourself steady.

3. Make sure you push your chest up and hips forward whilst holding the position for 20-30 seconds and repeat twice. You should feel a nice stretch in your quads.

4. Repeat using the left leg and right hand.

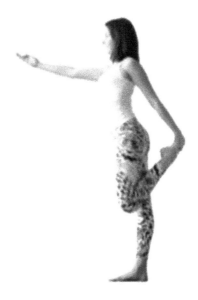

PIRIFORMIS

The piriformis is a small muscle located deep in the buttock, behind the gluteus maximus. The piriformis stretch feels as if you're stretching the gluteal (butt) muscles.

Piriformis and Outer Hip Stretch

1. Lie down on your back, place both feet flat on the floor and bend both knees.

2. Place your left ankle on (or just below) your right knee so that your left ankle is closer to you.

3. Grab your right knee with both hands and pull towards your chest. You will feel a stretch on the left gluteal muscle and back of the left leg when you do this.

4. Hold for 20-30 seconds and repeat twice.

5. Then repeat the above with the right leg.

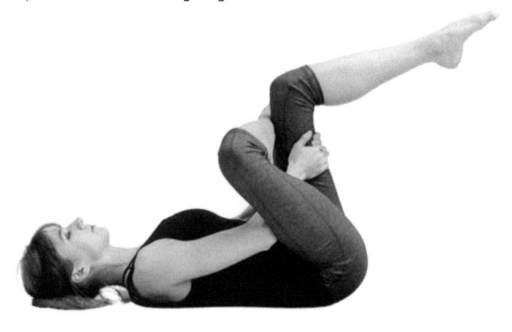

CALF MUSCLES

When the two main calf muscles (the gastrocnemius and the soleus) are tight and inflexible, they might affect your distribution of weight and the pressure you're applying to other areas of your body as you move around.

Simple Calf Stretch

1. Place one foot in front of the other, whilst the front knee is slightly bent.
   (Alternatively, stand in front of a wall and lean towards it.

2. Keep your back knee and leg straight, your heel on the ground, and lean forwards.

3. Slowly push until you feel a nice stretch inn the calf muscles.

4. Hold for 20-30 seconds, repeat twice and switch legs.

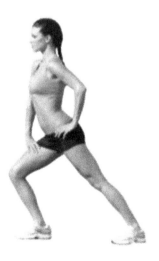

ADDUCTORS

The adductors, often referred to as your groin muscles, are a group of muscles that sit around your inner thigh area.

Standing Adductor Stretch

1. Stand with your feet approximately 3 feet apart.

2. Turn towards the right and bend your right knee whilst keeping the left leg straight until you feel a stretch in the inner part of your left thigh. Try to avoid your knee going in front of your toes.

3. Hold for 30 seconds, repeat twice.

4. Repeat the above steps with the left leg bent.

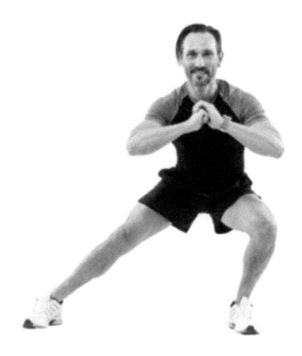

ABDOMINAL

The 'cobra pose' increases the flexibility of the spine. It stretches the chest while strengthening the spine and shoulders. It also helps to open the lungs and stretches the abdominal muscles.

Cobra Pose

1. Lie down on your stomach with your legs straight and the feet hip-width apart.

2. Press feet (nails down) into the floor and place palms on the ground next to your rib cage so that **your forearms are vertical**.

3. Inhale as you gently lift your head and chest off the floor. Keep your lower ribs on the floor.

4. Draw your shoulders back, do not crunch your neck. Keep your shoulders dropped away from your ears. Slowly push upwards until you feel an abdominal stretch.

5. Only straighten your arms as much as your body allows. Deepen the stretch as your practice advances, but avoid straining to achieve a deeper backbend. If your flexibility permits, you can straighten your arms all the way while maintaining the connection of the front of your pelvis and legs with the floor.

* **Caution**: Seek advice from your doctor if you have any 'back' problems when doing this stretch.

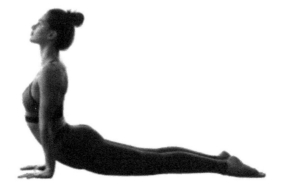

HIPS AND ILITIBIAL (IT) BAND

Your iliotibial band (IT band) is a thickened band of tissue that runs all the way down the length of your thigh. It helps stabilise your knees, but can become very inflamed and tight after prolonged running, cycling or leg exercises.

Seated Hip, Glute and ITB Stretch

1. Sit on the floor with both legs extended in front of you.

2. Cross the right leg over the left so that the right foot is flat on the floor.

3. Place your right hand on the floor behind your body as in the diagram.

4. Place your left hand on your outer right thigh. Alternatively, place your left elbow on the outside of your right knee (if you're flexible enough).

5. Pull your right leg to the left whilst twisting your torso to the right.

6. Hold for 30 seconds and repeat twice. Repeat the above steps using the left leg and the right arm to pull.

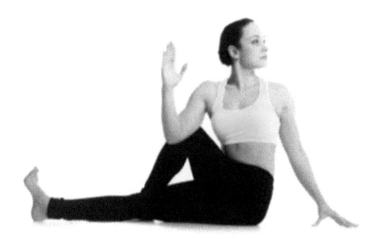

DELTOIDS

This exercise helps increase flexibility and range of motion in your shoulder joint and the surrounding muscles. When doing this exercise, lower your arm if you feel any pain in your shoulder.

Across-The-Chest Stretch

1. Straighten your right arm and extend your right arm across the chest so the biceps are touching the pecs.

2. Place your left hand onto the crease of the right elbow and pull further towards your chest.

3. Hold this position for 30 seconds.

4. Repeat on the other side.

5. Do each side 3 more times.

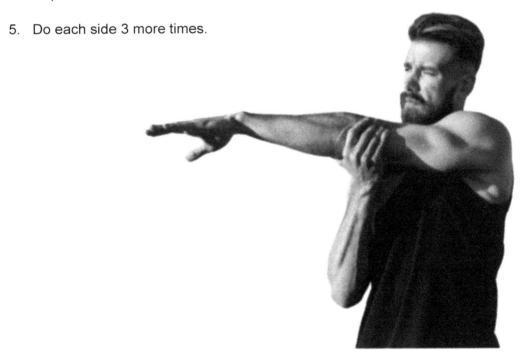

TRICEPS

The benefits of stretching the triceps are to improve flexibility and increase muscle length, improve function and maintain range of motion around elbows.

Across-The-Chest Stretch

1. Stand with your back straight and your feet shoulder-width apart. You can do this stretch sitting down if that's more comfortable for you.

2. Lift your right hand straight above your head and bend at the elbow. Keep your chin tucked in.

3. Place your left hand on your right elbow and gently pull down until you feel a stretch in the triceps.

4. Hold in this position for 30 seconds and repeat twice.

5. Switch arms remembering to keep your chin tucked in.

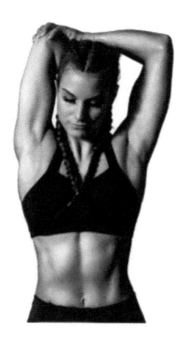

PECTORALIS & BICEPS

This is an excellent stretch following an upper body workout as it will relieve muscle tightness and tension in the biceps, chest and shoulder muscles.

Wall Bicep/Chest Stretch

1. Press your left palm against something sturdy like a wall or post.

2. Ensure your arm is straight and fingers are pointing away from you.

3. Slowly rotate your body away from the wall until you feel a stretch in your chest and biceps.

4. Hold this position for 30 seconds and repeat twice.

5. Switch arms.

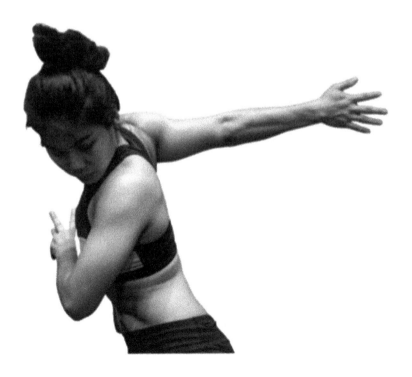

...IS THAT IT??

- You are probably aware of **other** stretches you can do and add to your routine, and I would strongly encourage you to do so.

- The above 10 stretches, however, will significantly reduce the risk of injury in the long term by keeping your muscles and joints flexible and supple.

- Remember to ideally reserve these stretches until after your workout once your muscles are already warm. This reduces the risk of potential injury, and we don't want that.

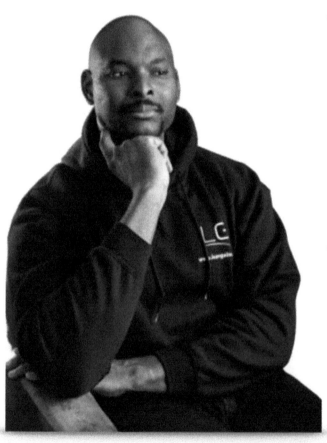

- However, as with the weight training and cardio sessions, you **must** see a physiotherapist or doctor if you start to feel any discomfort during or after your gym sessions. It's always better to tackle any potential problems early on since the longer you wait, the longer it takes to treat.

- Likewise, seek medical advice if you have any pre-existing injuries, heart problems, or any other medical condition, prior to undertaking any of the aforementioned workouts in this book. After all, prevention is always better than cure.

PART THREE

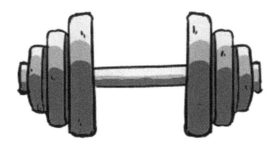

YOUR **NEW** GYM WORKOUT

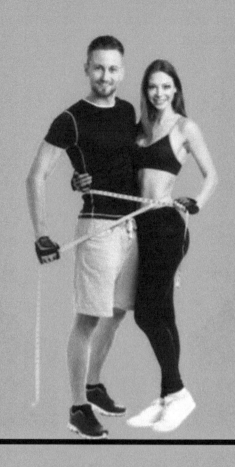

THE BEGINNER'S WORKOUT

THE 5-DAY WORKOUT FOR <u>MEN</u>

DAY	MAIN FOCUS
MONDAY	CHEST, LEGS & BACK
WEDNESDAY	BACK & SHOULDERS
FRIDAY	CHEST, LEGS & BACK
WEEKEND	REST

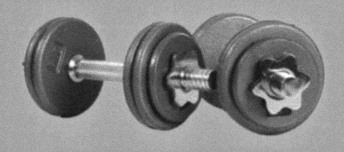

MONDAY

WARM UP

WARMUP SEQUENCE	REP RANGE	INTENSITY (%)	REST
LIGHT CARDIO	3 -5 MINUTES	30	
1ST WARMUP SET	10-12 REPS	50	1 minute
2ND WARMUP SET	10-12 REPS	50	1 minute
3RD WARMUP SET	4-6 REPS	70	1 minute
4TH WARMUP SET	1-2 REPS	90-95	3 minutes

MONDAY

THE BEGINNER'S WORKOUT

EXERCISE	SETS	REPS	REST
BENCH PRESS	3	8-12	1-2 minutes
FRONT SQUATS	3	8-12	1-2 minutes
ROWS	3	8-12	1-2 minutes

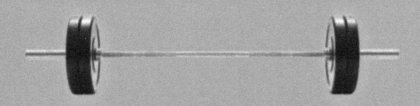

WEDNESDAY

THE BEGINNER'S WORKOUT

EXERCISE	SETS	REPS	REST
DEADLIFTS	3	8-12	1-2 minutes
LAT PULLDOWNS	3	8-12	1-2 minutes
MILITARY PRESS	3	8-12	1-2 minutes

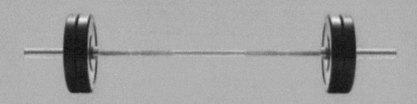

FRIDAY

<u>THE BEGINNER'S WORKOUT</u>

EXERCISE	SETS	REPS	REST
BENCH PRESS	3	8-12	1-2 minutes
BARBELL SQUATS	3	8-12	1-2 minutes
ROWS	3	8-12	1-2 minutes

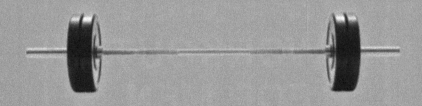

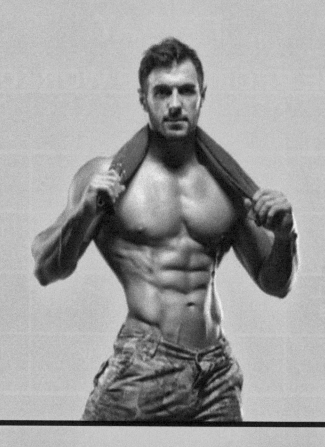

OPTION A

THE 5-DAY WORKOUT FOR MEN

THE 5-DAY WORKOUT FOR <u>MEN</u>

DAY	MAIN FOCUS
MONDAY	CHEST, LEGS & BACK
WEDNESDAY	BACK & SHOULDERS
WEDNESDAY	BACK & ABS
THURSDAY	SHOULDERS & CALVES
FRIDAY	CHEST, LEGS & BACK
WEEKEND	REST

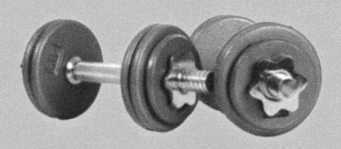

MONDAY

<u>WARM UP</u>

WARMUP SEQUENCE	REP RANGE	INTENSITY (%)	REST
LIGHT CARDIO	3 -5 MINUTES	30	
1ST WARMUP SET	10-12 REPS	50	1 minute
2ND WARMUP SET	10-12 REPS	50	1 minute
3RD WARMUP SET	4-6 REPS	70	1 minute
4TH WARMUP SET	1-2 REPS	90-95	3 minutes

MONDAY

<u>THE ESSENTIALS</u>

EXERCISE	SETS	REPS	REST
BARBELL SQUATS	3	4-6	3 minutes
FRONT SQUATS	3	4-6	3 minutes
HIP THRUSTS	3	6-8	3 minutes
ROMANIAN DEADLIFTS	3	4-6	3 minutes
SEATED/ STANDING CALF RAISES	3	8-10	1-2 minutes
DUMBBELL BICEP CURLS	3	4-6	3 minutes
BARBELL BICEP CURL	3	6-8	3 minutes

MONDAY

EXTRAS

**PICK 2-4 EXERCISES ONCE
YOU'VE DONE THE ESSENTIALS**

EXERCISE	SETS	REPS	REST
LEG CURL	3	8-12	1-2 minutes
LEG PRESS	3	8-12	1-2 minutes
DUMBBELL/ BARBELL LUNGE	3	8-12	1-2 minutes
HAMMER CURLS	3	8-12	1-2 minutes
CHIN UPS	3	FAILURE	1-2 minutes
CALF RAISES ON LEG PRESS	3	8-12	1-2 minutes

MONDAY

TRACK YOUR PROGRESS

USE THE BOXES BELOW TO TRACK YOUR
PROGRESS FOR THE 'ESSENTIAL' EXERCISES

EXERCISE	BARBELL SQUATS	FRONT SQUATS	ROMAN DEADLIFT	CALF RAISE	BICEP CURLS	E-Z BARBELL
WEEK 1						
WEEK 2						
WEEK 3						
WEEK 4						
WEEK5						
WEEK 6						
WEEK 7						
WEEK 8						
WEEK9						
WEEK10						
WEEK 11						
WEEK12						
WEEK 13						
WEEK 14						

TUESDAY

<u>WARM UP</u>

WARMUP SEQUENCE	REP RANGE	INTENSITY (%)	REST
LIGHT CARDIO	3 -5 MINUTES	30	
1ST WARMUP SET	10-12 REPS	50	1 minute
2ND WARMUP SET	10-12 REPS	50	1 minute
3RD WARMUP SET	4-6 REPS	70	1 minute
4TH WARMUP SET	1-2 REPS	90-95	3 minutes

TUESDAY

<u>THE ESSENTIALS</u>

EXERCISE	SETS	REPS	REST
FLAT BARBELL BENCH-PRESS	3	4-6	3 minutes
INCLINED DUMBBELL/ BARBELL BENCH PRESS	3	4-6	3 minutes
CLOSE-GRIP BENCH PRESS	3	4-6	3 minutes
SKULL CRUSHER	3	6-8	3 minutes
FACEPULL	3	8-12	1-2 minutes

TUESDAY

<u>EXTRAS</u>

PICK 2-4 EXERCISES ONCE
YOU'VE DONE THE ESSENTIALS

EXERCISE	SETS	REPS	REST
DIPS	3	8-10	1-2 minutes
DUMBBELL FLYES	3	8-10	1-2 minutes
DUMBBELL PULLOVER	3	8-10	1-2 minutes
TRICEP PRESS	3	8-12	1-2 minutes
TRICEPS PUSHDOWN	3	12-15	1-2 minutes
CABLE CROSSOVER	3	10-12	1-2 minutes
DUMBBELL FLYES	3	10-12	1-2 minutes
INTERNAL/ EXTERNAL DUMBBELL ROTATION	3	8-12	1-2 minutes

TUESDAY

TRACK YOUR PROGRESS

USE THE BOXES BELOW TO TRACK YOUR PROGRESS FOR THE 'ESSENTIAL' EXERCISES

EXERCISE	FLAT BARBELL BENCH PRESS	INCLINED DUMBBELL/ BARBELL BENCH PRESS	CLOSE-GRIP BENCH PRESS	SEATED TRICEP PRESS	FACEPULL
WEEK 1					
WEEK 2					
WEEK 3					
WEEK 4					
WEEK5					
WEEK 6					
WEEK 7					
WEEK 8					
WEEK9					
WEEK10					
WEEK 11					
WEEK12					
WEEK 13					
WEEK 14					

WEDNESDAY

<u>WARM UP</u>

WARMUP SEQUENCE	REP RANGE	INTENSITY (%)	REST
LIGHT CARDIO	3 -5 MINUTES	30	
1ST WARMUP SET	10-12 REPS	50	1 minute
2ND WARMUP SET	10-12 REPS	50	1 minute
3RD WARMUP SET	4-6 REPS	70	1 minute
4TH WARMUP SET	1-2 REPS	90-95	1 minute

WEDNESDAY

THE ESSENTIALS

EXERCISE	SETS	REPS	REST
BARBELL DEADLIFT	3	4-6	3 minutes
BARBELL ROW	3	4-6	3 minutes
WIDE-GRIP PULL UP	3	4-6	1 minutes
CABLE CRUNCH	3	4-6	1 minutes
HANGING LEG RAISES	3	TO FAILURE	1 minutes
AIR BIKE	3	TO FAILURE	1 minutes
AB ROLLERS	3	TO FAILURE	1 minutes

WEDNESDAY

<u>EXTRAS</u>

**PICK 2-4 EXERCISES ONCE
YOU'VE DONE THE ESSENTIALS**

EXERCISE	SETS	REPS	REST
ONE-ARM DUMBBELL ROW	3	8-10	1-2 minutes
BARBELL/ DUMBBELL SHRUG	3	8-12	3 minutes
LAT PULLDOWN	3	8-12	1-2 minutes
T-BAR ROW	3	8-12	1-2 minutes
HYPER-EXTENSION	3	8-12	1-2 minutes
LEG RAISES	3	10-12	1-2 minutes

WEDNESDAY

TRACK YOUR PROGRESS

USE THE BOXES BELOW TO TRACK YOUR
PROGRESS FOR THE 'ESSENTIAL' EXERCISES

EXERCISE	BARBELL DEADLIFT	BARBELL ROW	WIDE GRIP PULL UP	CABLE CRUNCH
WEEK 1				
WEEK 2				
WEEK 3				
WEEK 4				
WEEK5				
WEEK 6				
WEEK 7				
WEEK 8				
WEEK9				
WEEK10				
WEEK 11				
WEEK12				
WEEK 13				
WEEK 14				

THURSDAY

<u>WARM UP</u>

WARMUP SEQUENCE	REP RANGE	INTENSITY (%)	REST
LIGHT CARDIO	3 -5 MINUTES	30	
1ST WARMUP SET	10-12 REPS	50	1 minute
2ND WARMUP SET	10-12 REPS	50	1 minute
3RD WARMUP SET	4-6 REPS	70	1 minute
4TH WARMUP SET	1-2 REPS	90-95	3 minute

THURSDAY

<u>THE ESSENTIALS</u>

EXERCISE	SETS	REPS	REST
MILITARY PRESS	3	4-6	3 minutes
SIDE LATERAL RAISE	3	4-6	3 minutes
BARBELL REAR DELT ROW	3	4-6	3 minutes
CALF RAISES (STANDING/ SEATED)	3	4-6	3 minutes

THURSDAY

EXTRAS

**PICK 2-4 EXERCISES ONCE
YOU'VE DONE THE ESSENTIALS**

EXERCISE	SETS	REPS	REST
REAR DELT RAISE	3	8-12	1-2 minutes
ARNOLD DUMBBELL PRESS	3	10-15	1-2 minutes
DUMBBELL FRONT RAISE	3	8-12	1-2 minutes
BENT OVER DUMBBELL LATERAL RAISE	3	8-12	1-2 minutes
CALF RAISES ON LEG PRESS MACHINE	3	8-12	1-2 minutes

THURSDAY

TRACK YOUR PROGRESS

USE THE BOXES BELOW TO TRACK YOUR
PROGRESS FOR THE 'ESSENTIAL' EXERCISES

EXERCISE	MILITARY PRESS	SIDE LATERAL RAISE	BARBELL REAR DELT ROW	CALF RAISES
WEEK 1				
WEEK 2				
WEEK 3				
WEEK 4				
WEEK5				
WEEK 6				
WEEK 7				
WEEK 8				
WEEK9				
WEEK10				
WEEK 11				
WEEK12				
WEEK 13				
WEEK 14				

FRIDAY

<u>WARM UP</u>

WARMUP SEQUENCE	REP RANGE	INTENSITY (%)	REST
LIGHT CARDIO	3-5 MINUTES	30	

<u>The 'Friday' Workout</u>

It's ideal to train the same muscle groups at least twice per week. This is especially true with the smaller muscles such as the abs, biceps, etc.

However, in order to avoid injury or overtraining, the perspective working muscle should undergo one 'heavy' session (low-rep) and one 'lighter' session (higher rep) to maintain adequate growth.

The 'Friday' workout, in addition to the other routines highlighted above, allows for this to occur. As you can see, the 'Friday' sessions have a higher rep range, and hence relatively lighter weights are indicated here.

FRIDAY

<u>WHOLE BODY</u>

EXERCISE	SETS	REPS	REST
DUMBBELL PULLOVER	3	8-12	2 minutes
LEG PRESS	3	8-12	2 minutes
HAMMER CURL	3	8-12	2 minutes
HYPER EXTENSION	3	8-12	2 minutes
TRICEPS PUSHDOWN	3	8-12	2 minutes
FACEPULL	3	8-12	2 minutes
CAPTAIN CHAIR LEG RAISE	3	8-12	1-2 minutes
AIR BICYCLES	3	TO FAILURE	1 minutes
AB ROLLER	3	TO FAILURE	1 minutes

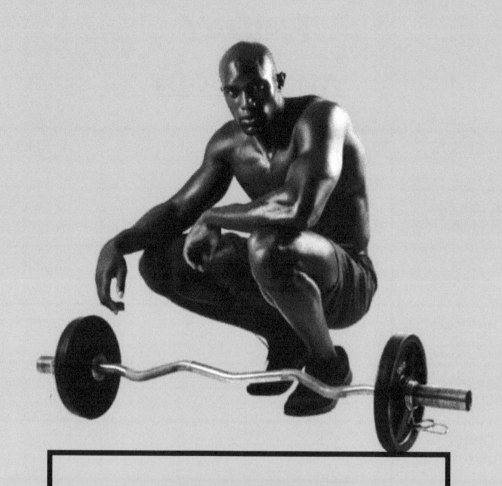

OPTION B

THE 3-DAY WORKOUT FOR ME

THE 3-DAY WORKOUT
FOR <u>MEN</u>

DAY	MAIN FOCUS
MONDAY	BACK, ABS & BICEPS
WEDNESDAY	CHEST, TRICEPS & CALVES
FRIDAY	LEGS & SHOULDERS
WEEKEND	REST

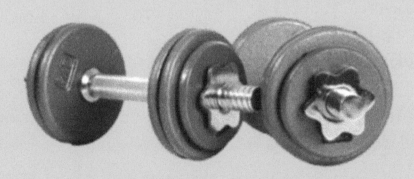

MONDAY

<u>WARM UP</u>

WARMUP SEQUENCE	REP RANGE	INTENSITY (%)	REST
LIGHT CARDIO	3 -5 MINUTES	30	
1ST WARMUP SET	10-12 REPS	50	1 minute
2ND WARMUP SET	10-12 REPS	50	1 minute
3RD WARMUP SET	4-6 REPS	70	1 minute
4TH WARMUP SET	1-2 REPS	90-95	3 minute

MONDAY

THE ESSENTIALS

EXERCISE	SETS	REPS	REST
DEADLIFT	3	4-6	3 minutes
BARBELL ROW	3	4-6	3 minutes
PULL UPS	3	4-6	3 minutes
BICEP CURLS	3	8-10	3 minutes
HANGING LEG RAISES [weighted if possible]	3	10-12	1-2 minutes
CABLE CRUNCH	3	10-12	1 minute
AIR BICYCLES	3	TO FAILURE	1 minute

MONDAY

EXTRAS

**PICK 2-4 EXERCISES ONCE
YOU'VE DONE THE ESSENTIALS**

EXERCISE	SETS	REPS	REST
BARBELLL SHRUG	3	8-12	1-2 minutes
HYPER EXTENSION	3	8-12	1-2 minutes
HAMMER CURLS	3	8-12	1-2 minutes
BENT OVER DUMBBELL LATERAL RAISE	3	8-12	1-2 minutes
LAT PULLDOWN	3	12-15	1-2 minutes

MONDAY

TRACK YOUR PROGRESS

USE THE BOXES BELOW TO TRACK YOUR
PROGRESS FOR THE 'ESSENTIAL' EXERCISES

EXERCISE	DEADLIFTS	BARBELL ROW	BICEP CURLS	HANGING LEG RAISES WEIGHTED	CABLE CRUNCH
WEEK 1					
WEEK 2					
WEEK 3					
WEEK 4					
WEEK5					
WEEK 6					
WEEK 7					
WEEK 8					
WEEK9					
WEEK10					
WEEK 11					
WEEK12					
WEEK 13					
WEEK 14					

WEDNESDAY

<u>WARM UP</u>

WARMUP SEQUENCE	REP RANGE	INTENSITY (%)	REST
LIGHT CARDIO	3 -5 MINUTES	30	
1ST WARMUP SET	10-12 REPS	50	1 minute
2ND WARMUP SET	10-12 REPS	50	1 minute
3RD WARMUP SET	4-6 REPS	70	1 minute
4TH WARMUP SET	1-2 REPS	90-95	3 minute

WEDNESDAY

THE ESSENTIALS

EXERCISE	SETS	REPS	REST
BENCH PRESS	3	4-6	3 minutes
INCLINED DUMBBELL PRESS	3	4-6	3 minutes
SKULL CRUSHERS	3	4-6	3 minutes
CALF RAISES (Standed/ Seated)	3	4-6	3 minutes

WEDNESDAY

EXTRAS

**PICK 2-4 EXERCISES ONCE
YOU'VE DONE THE ESSENTIALS**

EXERCISE	SETS	REPS	REST
DUMBBELL PULLOVER	3	8-12	1-2 minutes
DIPS	3	8-12	1-2 minutes
CABLE CROSSOVER	3	10-15	1-2 minutes
TRICEPS PUSHDOWN	3	8-12	1-2 minutes
CLOSE-GRIP BENCH PRESS	3	10-15	1-2 minutes
CALF RAISES ON LEG PRESS	3	10-15	1-2 minutes

WEDNESDAY

TRACK YOUR PROGRESS

USE THE BOXES BELOW TO TRACK YOUR
PROGRESS FOR THE 'ESSENTIAL' EXERCISES

EXERCISE	BENCH PRESS	INCLINED DUMBBELL	SEATED TRICEP PRESS	CALF RAISES
WEEK 1				
WEEK 2				
WEEK 3				
WEEK 4				
WEEK5				
WEEK 6				
WEEK 7				
WEEK 8				
WEEK9				
WEEK10				
WEEK 11				
WEEK12				
WEEK 13				
WEEK 14				

FRIDAY

<u>WARM UP</u>

WARMUP SEQUENCE	REP RANGE	INTENSITY (%)	REST
LIGHT CARDIO	3-5 MINUTES	30	
1ST WARMUP SET	10-12 REPS	50	1 minute
2ND WARMUP SET	10-12 REPS	50	1 minute
3RD WARMUP SET	4-6 REPS	70	1 minute
4TH WARMUP SET	1-2 REPS	90-95	3 minute

FRIDAY

<u>THE ESSENTIALS</u>

EXERCISE	SETS	REPS	REST
BARBELL SQUATS	3	4-6	3 minutes
FRONT SQUATS	3	4-6	3 minutes
ROMANIAN DEADLIFT	3	4-6	3 minutes
MILITARY PRESS	3	4-6	3 minutes
BARBELL REAR DELT ROW	3	4-6	3 minutes

FRIDAY

EXTRAS

**PICK 2-4 EXERCISES ONCE
YOU'VE DONE THE ESSENTIALS**

EXERCISE	SETS	REPS	REST
LEG PRESS	3	8-12	1-2 minutes
DUMBBELL/ BARBELL LUNGES	3	8-12	1-2 minutes
DUMBBELL FRONT RAISES	3	10-15	1-2 minutes
ARNOLD DUMBBELL PRESS	3	8-12	1-2 minutes
DUMBBELL SIDE LATERAL RAISES	3	10-15	1-2 minutes
REAR DELT RAISE	3	10-15	1-2 minutes

FRIDAY

TRACK YOUR PROGRESS

USE THE BOXES BELOW TO TRACK YOUR
PROGRESS FOR THE 'ESSENTIAL' EXERCISES

EXERCISE	BARBELL SQUATS	FRONT SQUATS	ROMANIAN DEADLIFTS	MILITARY PRESS	BARBELL REAR DELT ROW
WEEK 1					
WEEK 2					
WEEK 3					
WEEK 4					
WEEK 5					
WEEK 6					
WEEK 7					
WEEK 8					
WEEK 9					
WEEK 10					
WEEK 11					
WEEK 12					
WEEK 13					
WEEK 14					

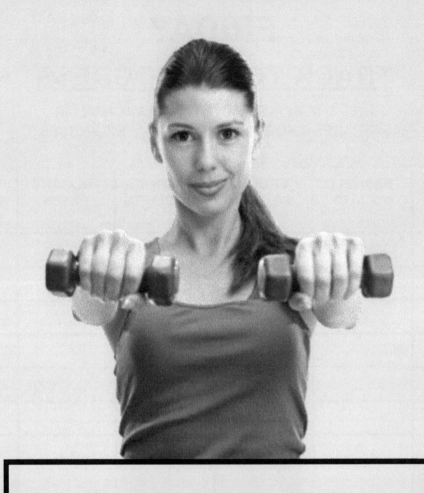

OPTION A

THE 5-DAY WORKOUT FOR WOMEN

THE 3-DAY WORKOUT
FOR <u>WOMEN</u>

DAY	MAIN FOCUS
MONDAY	LEGS & BICEPS
TUESDAY	CHEST & TRICEPS
WEDNESDAY	BACK, BUTT & ABS
THURSDAY	SHOULDERS & CALVES
FRIDAY	WHOLE BODY
WEEKEND	REST

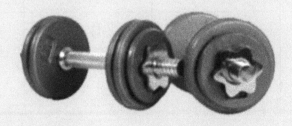

MONDAY

WARM UP

WARMUP SEQUENCE	REP RANGE	INTENSITY (%)	REST
LIGHT CARDIO	3 -5 MINUTES	30	
1ST WARMUP SET	10-12 REPS	50	1 minute
2ND WARMUP SET	10-12 REPS	50	1 minute
3RD WARMUP SET	4-6 REPS	70	1 minute
4TH WARMUP SET	1-2 REPS	90-95	3 minute

MONDAY

<u>THE ESSENTIALS</u>

EXERCISE	SETS	REPS	REST
BARBELL SQUATS	3	4-6	3 minutes
FRONT SQUATS	3	4-6	3 minutes
ROMANIAN DEADLIFTS	3	4-6	3 minutes
HIP THRUST	3	4-8	3 minutes
CALVES RAISES (SEATED/ STANDING)	3	8-10	1-2 minutes

MONDAY

EXTRAS

**PICK 2-4 EXERCISES ONCE
YOU'VE DONE THE ESSENTIALS**

EXERCISE	SETS	REPS	REST
LEGCURL	3	8-12	1-2 minutes
LEGPRESS	3	8-12	1-2 minutes
DUMBBEL/ BARBELL LUNGE	3	8-12	1-2 minutes
BUTT BLASTER/ GLUTE MASTER	3	8-12	1-2 minutes
CALF RAISES ON LEG PRESS MACHINE	3	8-12	1-2 minutes

MONDAY

TRACK YOUR PROGRESS

USE THE BOXES BELOW TO TRACK YOUR
PROGRESS FOR THE 'ESSENTIAL' EXERCISES

EXERCISE	BARBELL SQUATS	FRONT SQUATS	ROMAN DEADLIFT	HIP THRUST	SEATED CALF RAISES
WEEK 1					
WEEK 2					
WEEK 3					
WEEK 4					
WEEK5					
WEEK 6					
WEEK 7					
WEEK 8					
WEEK9					
WEEK10					
WEEK 11					
WEEK12					
WEEK 13					
WEEK 14					

TUESDAY

WARM UP

WARMUP SEQUENCE	REP RANGE	INTENSITY (%)	REST
LIGHT CARDIO	3 -5 MINUTES	30	
1ST WARMUP SET	10-12 REPS	50	1 minute
2ND WARMUP SET	10-12 REPS	50	1 minute
3RD WARMUP SET	4-6 REPS	70	1 minute
4TH WARMUP SET	1-2 REPS	90-95	3 minute

TUESDAY

THE ESSENTIALS

EXERCISE	SETS	REPS	REST
FLAT BARBELL BENCHPRESS	3	4-6	3 minutes
INCLINED DUMBBELL/ BARBELL BENCH PRESS	3	4-6	3 minutes
CLOSE-GRIP BENCH PRESS	3	4-6	3 minutes
SKULL CRUSHERS	3	4-8	3 minutes
FACEPULL	3	8-12	1-2 minutes

TUESDAY

EXTRAS

**PICK 2-4 EXERCISES ONCE
YOU'VE DONE THE ESSENTIALS**

EXERCISE	SETS	REPS	REST
DIPS	3	8-10	1-2 minutes
DUMBBELL FLYES	3	8-10	1-2 minutes
DUMBBELL PULLOVER	3	8-10	1-2 minutes
TRICEP PRESS	3	8-12	1-2 minutes
TRICEPS PUSHDOWN	3	12-15	1-2 minutes
CABLE CROSSOVER	3	10-12	1-2 minutes
DUMBBELL FLYES	3	10-12	1-2 minutes
INTERNAL/ EXTERNAL DUMBBELL ROTATION	3	8-12	1-2 minutes

TUESDAY

TRACK YOUR PROGRESS

USE THE BOXES BELOW TO TRACK YOUR
PROGRESS FOR THE 'ESSENTIAL' EXERCISES

EXERCISE	FLAT BARBELL BENCH PRESS	INCLINED DUMBBELL/ BARBELL BENCH PRESS	CLOSE-GRIP BENCH PRESS	SEATED TRICEP PRESS	FACEPULL
WEEK 1					
WEEK 2					
WEEK 3					
WEEK 4					
WEEK5					
WEEK 6					
WEEK 7					
WEEK 8					
WEEK9					
WEEK10					
WEEK 11					
WEEK12					
WEEK 13					
WEEK 14					

WEDNESDAY

<u>WARM UP</u>

WARMUP SEQUENCE	REP RANGE	INTENSITY (%)	REST
LIGHT CARDIO	3 -5 MINUTES	30	
1ST WARMUP SET	10-12 REPS	50	1 minute
2ND WARMUP SET	10-12 REPS	50	1 minute
3RD WARMUP SET	4-6 REPS	70	1 minute
4TH WARMUP SET	1-2 REPS	90-95	3 minute

WEDNESDAY

THE ESSENTIALS

EXERCISE	SETS	REPS	REST
BARBELL DEADLIFT	3	4-6	3 minutes
BARBELL ROW	3	4-6	3 minutes
WIDE-GRIP PULL UP	3	4-6	3 minutes
CABLE CRUNCH	3	10-12	1 minute
HANGING LEG RAISES	3	TO FAILURE	1 minute
AIR BIKE	3	TO FAILURE	1 minute
AB ROLLERS	3	TO FAILURE	1 minute

WEDNESDAY

<u>EXTRAS</u>

**PICK 2-4 EXERCISES ONCE
YOU'VE DONE THE ESSENTIALS**

EXERCISE	SETS	REPS	REST
ONE-ARM DUMBBELL ROW	3	8-10	1-2 minutes
BARBELL/ DUMBBELL SHRUG	3	8-12	3 minutes
LAT PULLDOWN	3	8-12	1-2 minutes
T-BAR ROW	3	8-12	1-2 minutes
HYPER- EXTENSION	3	8-12	1-2 minutes
LEG RAISES	3	TO FAILURE	1-2 minutes

WEDNESDAY

TRACK YOUR PROGRESS

USE THE BOXES BELOW TO TRACK YOUR
PROGRESS FOR THE 'ESSENTIAL' EXERCISES

EXERCISE	FLAT BARBELL BENCH PRESS	INCLINED DUMBBELL/ BARBELL BENCH PRESS	CLOSE-GRIP BENCH PRESS	SEATED TRICEP PRESS
WEEK 1				
WEEK 2				
WEEK 3				
WEEK 4				
WEEK5				
WEEK 6				
WEEK 7				
WEEK 8				
WEEK9				
WEEK10				
WEEK 11				
WEEK12				
WEEK 13				
WEEK 14				

THURSDAY

WARM UP

WARMUP SEQUENCE	REP RANGE	INTENSITY (%)	REST
LIGHT CARDIO	3 -5 MINUTES	30	
1ST WARMUP SET	10-12 REPS	50	1 minute
2ND WARMUP SET	10-12 REPS	50	1 minute
3RD WARMUP SET	4-6 REPS	70	1 minute
4TH WARMUP SET	1-2 REPS	90-95	3 minute

THURSDAY

THE ESSENTIALS

EXERCISE	SETS	REPS	REST
MILITARY PRESS	3	4-6	3 minutes
SIDE LATERAL RAISE	3	4-6	3 minutes
BARBELL REAR DELT ROW	3	4-6	3 minutes
CALF RAISES (STANDING/ SEATED)	3	4-6	3 minutes

THURSDAY

<u>EXTRAS</u>

**PICK 2-4 EXERCISES ONCE
YOU'VE DONE THE ESSENTIALS**

EXERCISE	SETS	REPS	REST
REAR DELT RAISE	3	8-12	1-2 minutes
ARNOLD DUMBBELL PRESS	3	10-15	1-2 minutes
DUMBBELL FRONT RAISE	3	8-12	1-2 minutes
BENT OVER DUMBBELL LATERAL RAISE	3	8-12	1-2 minutes
CALF RAISES ON LEG PRESS MACHINE	3	12-15	1-2 minutes

THURSDAY

TRACK YOUR PROGRESS

USE THE BOXES BELOW TO TRACK YOUR
PROGRESS FOR THE 'ESSENTIAL' EXERCISES

EXERCISE	MILITARY PRESS	SIDE LATERAL RAISE	BARBELL REAR DELT ROW	CALF RAISES
WEEK 1				
WEEK 2				
WEEK 3				
WEEK 4				
WEEK5				
WEEK 6				
WEEK 7				
WEEK 8				
WEEK9				
WEEK10				
WEEK 11				
WEEK12				
WEEK 13				
WEEK 14				

FRIDAY

WARM UP

WARMUP SEQUENCE	REP RANGE	INTENSITY (%)	REST
LIGHT CARDIO	3-5 MINUTES	30	

The 'Friday' Workout

It's ideal to train the same muscle groups at least twice per week. This is especially true with the smaller muscles such as the abs, biceps, etc.

However, in order to avoid injury or overtraining, the perspective working muscle should undergo one 'heavy' session (low-rep) and one 'lighter' session (higher rep) to maintain adequate growth.

The 'Friday' workout, in addition to the other routines highlighted above, allows for this to occur. As you can see, the 'Friday' sessions have a higher rep range, and hence relatively lighter weights are indicated here.

FRIDAY
WHOLE BODY

EXERCISE	SETS	REPS	REST
SQUATS	3	8-12	2 minutes
LEG PRESS	3	8-12	2 minutes
HAMMER CURL	3	8-12	2 minutes
HYPER EXTENSION	3	8-12	2 minutes
TRICEP PUSHDOWN	3	8-12	2 minutes
FACEPULL	3	8-12	2 minutes
CAPTAIN CHAIR LEG RAISE	3	8-12	1-2 minutes
AIR BICYCLES	3	TO FAILURE	1 minute
AB ROLLER	3	TO FAILURE	1 minute

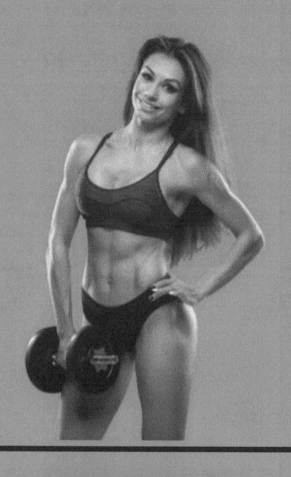

OPTION B

THE 3-DAY WORKOUT FOR WOMEN

THE 3-DAY WORKOUT
FOR <u>WOMEN</u>

DAY	MAIN FOCUS
MONDAY	BACK, BUTT & ABS
WEDNESDAY	CHEST, TRICEPS & CALVES
FRIDAY	LEGS, BUTT & SHOULDERS
WEEKEND	REST

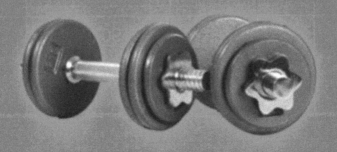

MONDAY

WARM UP

WARMUP SEQUENCE	REP RANGE	INTENSITY (%)	REST
LIGHT CARDIO	3-5 MINUTES	30	
1ST WARMUP SET	10-12 REPS	50	1 minute
2ND WARMUP SET	10-12 REPS	50	1 minute
3RD WARMUP SET	4-6 REPS	70	1 minute
4TH WARMUP SET	1-2 REPS	90-95	3 minutes

MONDAY

THE ESSENTIALS

EXERCISE	SETS	REPS	REST
DEADLIFTS	3	4-6	3 minutes
BARBELL ROW	3	4-6	3 minutes
PULL UPS	3	4-6	3 minutes
BICEP CURLS	3	8-10	3 minutes
BULGARIAN SPLIT SQUATS	3	10-12	1-2 minutes
CABLE CRUNCH	3	10-12	1 minute
AIR BICYCLES	3	TO FAILURE	1 minute

MONDAY

EXTRAS

**PICK 2-4 EXERCISES ONCE
YOU'VE DONE THE ESSENTIALS**

EXERCISE	SETS	REPS	REST
BARBELLL SHRUG	3	8-12	1-2 minutes
HYPER EXTENSION	3	8-12	1-2 minutes
HAMMER CURLS	3	8-12	1-2 minutes
BENT OVER DUMBBELL LATERAL RAISES	3	8-12	1-2 minutes
LAT PULLDOWN	3	12-15	1-2 minutes

MONDAY

TRACK YOUR PROGRESS

USE THE BOXES BELOW TO TRACK YOUR
PROGRESS FOR THE 'ESSENTIAL' EXERCISES

EXERCISE	DEADLIFTS	BARBELL ROW	BICEP CURLS	BULGARIAN SPLIT SQUATS	CABLE CRUNCH
WEEK 1					
WEEK 2					
WEEK 3					
WEEK 4					
WEEK 5					
WEEK 6					
WEEK 7					
WEEK 8					
WEEK 9					
WEEK 10					
WEEK 11					
WEEK 12					
WEEK 13					
WEEK 14					

WEDNESDAY

<u>WARM UP</u>

WARMUP SEQUENCE	REP RANGE	INTENSITY (%)	REST
LIGHT CARDIO	3-5 MINUTES	30	
1ST WARMUP SET	10-12 REPS	50	1 minute
2ND WARMUP SET	10-12 REPS	50	1 minute
3RD WARMUP SET	4-6 REPS	70	1 minute
4TH WARMUP SET	1-2 REPS	90-95	3 minute

WEDNESDAY

<u>THE ESSENTIALS</u>

EXERCISE	SETS	REPS	REST
BENCH PRESS	3	4-6	3 minutes
INCLINED DUMBBELL PRESS	3	4-6	3 minutes
SEATED TRICEP PRESS	3	4-6	3 minutes
CALF RAISES (STANDING/ SEATED)	3	4-6	3 minutes

WEDNESDAY

EXTRAS

PICK 2-4 EXERCISES ONCE
YOU'VE DONE THE ESSENTIALS

EXERCISE	SETS	REPS	REST
DUMBBELL PULLOVER	3	8-12	1-2 minutes
DIPS	3	8-12	1-2 minutes
CABLE CROSSOVER	3	10-15	1-2 minutes
TRICEPS PUSHDOWN	3	8-12	1-2 minutes
CLOSE-GRIP BENCH PRESS	3	10-15	1-2 minutes
CALF RAISES ON LEG PRESS	3	10-15	1-2 minutes

WEDNESDAY

TRACK YOUR PROGRESS

USE THE BOXES BELOW TO TRACK YOUR
PROGRESS FOR THE 'ESSENTIAL' EXERCISES

EXERCISE	BENCH PRESS	INCLINED DUMBBELL	SEATED TRICEP PRESS	CALF RAISES
WEEK 1				
WEEK 2				
WEEK 3				
WEEK 4				
WEEK 5				
WEEK 6				
WEEK 7				
WEEK 8				
WEEK 9				
WEEK 10				
WEEK 11				
WEEK 12				
WEEK 13				
WEEK 14				

FRIDAY

<u>WARM UP</u>

WARMUP SEQUENCE	REP RANGE	INTENSITY (%)	REST
LIGHT CARDIO	3-5 MINUTES	30	
1ST WARMUP SET	10-12 REPS	50	1 minute
2ND WARMUP SET	10-12 REPS	50	1 minute
3RD WARMUP SET	4-6 REPS	70	1 minute
4TH WARMUP SET	1-2 REPS	90-95	3 minute

FRIDAY

THE ESSENTIALS

EXERCISE	SETS	REPS	REST
BARBELL SQUATS	3	4-6	3 minutes
FRONT SQUATS	3	4-6	3 minutes
ROMANIAN DEADLIFT	3	4-6	3 minutes
HIP THRUST	3	4-6	3 minutes
MILITARY PRESS	3	4-6	3 minutes

FRIDAY

<u>EXTRAS</u>

**PICK 2-4 EXERCISES ONCE
YOU'VE DONE THE ESSENTIALS**

EXERCISE	SETS	REPS	REST
LEG PRESS	3	8-12	1-2 minutes
DUMBBELL/ BARBELL LUNGES	3	8-12	1-2 minutes
DUMBBELL FRONT RAISES	3	10-15	1-2 minutes
ARNOLD DUMBBELL PRESS	3	8-12	1-2 minutes
DUMBBELL SIDE LATERAL RAISES	3	10-15	1-2 minutes
REAR DELT RAISE	3	10-15	1-2 minutes

FRIDAY

TRACK YOUR PROGRESS

USE THE BOXES BELOW TO TRACK YOUR
PROGRESS FOR THE 'ESSENTIAL' EXERCISES

EXERCISE	BARBELL SQUATS	FRONT SQUATS	ROMANIAN DEADLIFTS	HIP THRUST	MILITARY PRESS
WEEK 1					
WEEK 2					
WEEK 3					
WEEK 4					
WEEK 5					
WEEK 6					
WEEK 7					
WEEK 8					
WEEK 9					
WEEK 10					
WEEK 11					
WEEK 12					
WEEK 13					
WEEK 14					

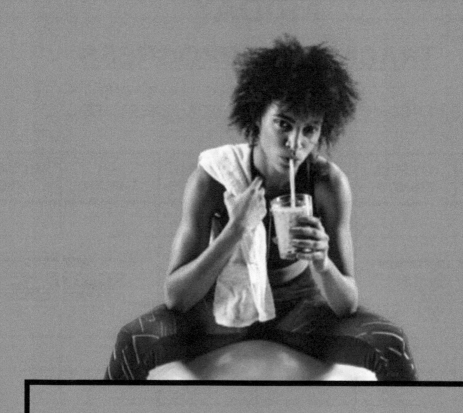

DELOAD
WEEK

DELOAD WEEK

TO BE DONE APPROXIMATELY
EVERY 8 WEEKS

DAY	MAIN FOCUS
MONDAY	DELOAD DAY 1
WEDNESDAY	DELOAD DAY 2
FRIDAY	DELOAD DAY 3
WEEKEND	DELOAD DAY 4

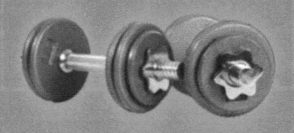

DELOAD WEEK

<u>WARM UP</u>

WARMUP SEQUENCE	REP RANGE	INTENSITY (%)	REST
LIGHT CARDIO	3-5 MINUTES	30	
1ST WARMUP SET	10-12 REPS	50	1 minute
2ND WARMUP SET	10-12 REPS	50	1 minute
3RD WARMUP SET	4-6 REPS	70	1 minute
4TH WARMUP SET	1-2 REPS	90-95	3 minute

MONDAY

DELOAD DAY 1

EXERCISE	SETS	REPS	REST
DEADLIFTS	3	8-12	3 minutes
BARBELL ROW	3	8-12	3 minutes
HANGING LEG RAISES	3	10-12	3 minutes
AB ROLLERS	3	8-12	3 minutes
BULGARIAN SPLIT SQUATS	3	10-12	3 minutes
AIR BICYCLES	3	10-12	2 minutes
AB ROLLERS	3	10-12	2 minutes

WEDNESDAY

DELOAD DAY 2

EXERCISE	SETS	REPS	REST
BENCH PRESS	3	8-12	3 minutes
INCLINED DUMBBELL PRESS	3	8-12	3 minutes
MILITARY PRESS	3	10-12	3 minutes

FRIDAY

<u>DELOAD DAY 3</u>

EXERCISE	SETS	REPS	REST
BARBELL SQUATS	3	8-12	3 minutes
FRONT SQUAT	3	8-12	3 minutes
ROMANIAN DEADLIFT	3	8-12	3 minutes
BARBELL CURLS	3	8-12	3 minutes

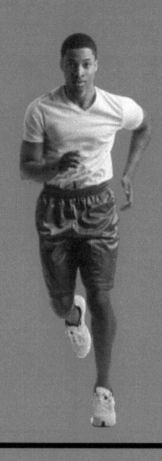

WHAT ABOUT CARDIO?

HOW TO ADD CARDIO TO YOUR WEEKLY ROUTINE

What is Cardio?

Cardiovascular Exercise (or cardio) is any activity that increases heart rate and respiration while using large muscle groups repetitively and rhythmically.

The main reason we do cardio is to help us keep fit and healthy, optimise heart function, and, above all, help us burn more calories (fat).

When it comes to building new muscle and getting ripped, however, cardio is no substitute to the aforementioned training regimes.

There are 3 main types of cardio that you can implement into your regime. They are:

- Low-Intensity Cardio
- High-Intensity Intermittent Training (HIIT)
- Metabolice Resistance Training (MRT)

LOW-INTENSITY
CARDIO

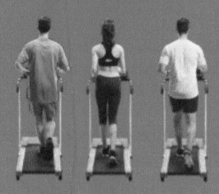

What is Low-Intensity Cardio?

Low-intensity cardio is when you perform low-impact exercises that fulfil all of the cardiovascular benefits of exercise without over-taxing the body.

Examples

Walking, Jogging, Swimming, Rowing, Walking or Light Jogging on a Treadmill, Bike-Riding, etc.

Duration and Frequency

45-60 minutes per session 2 times per week in addition to your weight training regimes should suffice.

HIGH-INTENSITY CARDIO

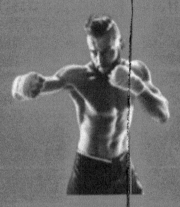

What is HIIT Cardio?

HIIT involves short bursts of intense exercise alternated with low-intensity or recovery periods.

Examples

Boxing, Sprinting, Skipping, Shaun T's Insanity Workout, Circuit Training, etc. HIIT sessions-1 and 2 on the following pages are also great HIIT exercises.

Duration and Frequency

20-30 minutes per session 2-3 times per week in addition to your weight training regimes should suffice.

HIIT SESSION-1

30-SECOND SPRINTS IN A
20 MINUTE HIIT SESSION

EXERCISE	DURATION
WARM-UP (eg. Light jog)	5 minutes
1st SPRINT	30 seconds
Walk/Light Jog	2 minutes
2nd SPRINT	30 seconds
Walk/Light Jog	2 minutes
3rd SPRINT	30 seconds
Walk/Light Jog	2 minutes
4th SPRINT	30 seconds
Walk/Light Jog	2 minutes
5th SPRINT	30 seconds
Walk/Light Jog	2 minutes
6th SPRINT	30 seconds
Cool down/stretch	5 minutes

HIIT SESSION-2

CIRCUIT TRAINING

WHAT IS CIRCUIT TRAINING?

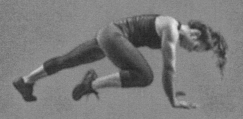

Circuit training is a fast-paced series of exercises whereby you do exercise from around 30-seconds to 2-minutes and then move onto another exercise.

EXERCISE	DURATION
WARM-UP (eg. Light jog)	5 minutes
BURPEES	30 seconds
JUMPING JACKS	30 seconds
SKIPPING	30 seconds
MOUNTAIN CLIMBERS	30 seconds
REST	30 seconds

WHAT ABOUT MRT?

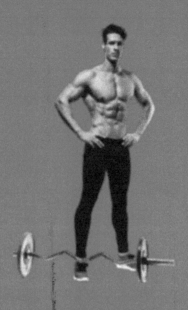

What is MRT?

MRT involves performing resistance and compound exercises at a very rapid pace with little or no rest in between exercises.

What Are The Protocols for MRT?

A Light Weight, Engaging All Muscle Groups (ie. Compound Exercises), and Short Rest Periods (between circuits).

Duration and Frequency

20-30 minutes per session no more than 2 times per week in addition to your weight training regimes should suffice.

A SAMPLE MRT CIRCUIT

HOW TO PERFORM THIS CIRCUIT?

Always start off with a 5-minute light jog. Then using a light-weight (eg. RPE 4), perform the following exercises without rest. Once you've finished the circuit, rest for 2 minutes. Repeat the circuit 5 more times.

EXERCISE	DURATION/REPS
WARM-UP (eg. Light jog)	5 minutes
BENCH PRESS	20 reps
DEADLIFT	20 reps
PULL-UPS	10 reps
OVERHEAD PRESS	20 reps
SQUATS	20 reps
REST	2 minutes

PART FOUR

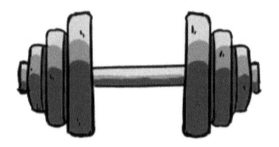

SOME
FREQUENTLY
ASKED

QUESTIONS

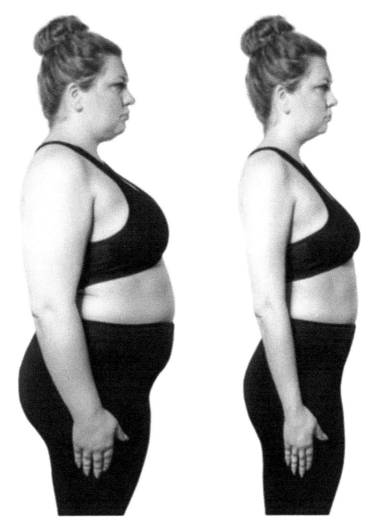

WHAT WILL I LOOK LIKE IN <u>10 WEEKS</u> IF I FOLLOW THIS WORKOUT PROGRAMME?

…NOW THAT'S A DAM GOOD QUESTION!!…

Let me start off by saying **first and foremost** that

THIS STUFF WORKS!!!!

There are **literally thousands of studies, papers, books and testimonials** that back up the science behind these workouts so there really is no need to look elsewhere for a more effective workout plan.

If you would like to learn more about the science behind them and how/why these workouts are so effective, then I would strongly suggest checking out my other book **'The Essential Guide to Sports Nutrition and Bodybuilding,'** and/or **'Lean Gains** (2nd Edition). Alternatively, feel free to take a look at the many references at the back of these books (as well as this book) so you can see for yourself.

Before answering this very common question, however, let me also say that you probably won't be satisfied with your results if your **diet is out of whack**. I go over diet in immense detail in **'The Essential Guide to Sports Nutrition and Bodybuilding.'** I have also recently written a recipe book **'Lean Meals for Everyone'** that contains **a wide range of tasty meal plans** that will make your 'fat-burning/muscle-building journey' more enjoyable.

Please visit **www.leangains.co.uk** for more information.

...ANYWAY, IN ANSWER
TO THE QUESTION...

...I REALLY DO NOT KNOW!!!!...

We all come in different shapes and sizes, so for that reason, it's unfair to make blanket promises as if there's a **one-size fits all solution** (pardon the pun).

In other words, it's going to take much longer for a guy who weighs 20 stone, has never been to the gym before and carries 35% body fat to look lean than another guy who's say 20% body fat.

That is why if you meet or come across anybody trying to sell you some random fitness product or service by saying any of the following:

- ❖ **Miracle drug** 'Fat-Off Now XYZ' will get you a 6-pack in 2 weeks!!

- ❖ **Revolutionary diet** that will enable you to drop 5 dress-sizes in 5 days!!

- ❖ **Incredible muscle-building** powder 'Muscle Grow-Rapid 1234' will get you to pack on 10 pounds of pure muscle in 1 month!!

- ❖ Brand New **Fitness Programme** 'Burn-Fat-Burn-ABCD' has doctors world-wide truly baffled. Start today and lose all your belly fat in 7 days!

- ❖ **Amy struggled with diets** in the past but has managed to drop 2 stone of weight in 5 weeks. She has got her friends to also drop 2 stones in weight by just following the 'get-ripped-and-tonedquick without-starving' diet!!

....then please do me this one favour....

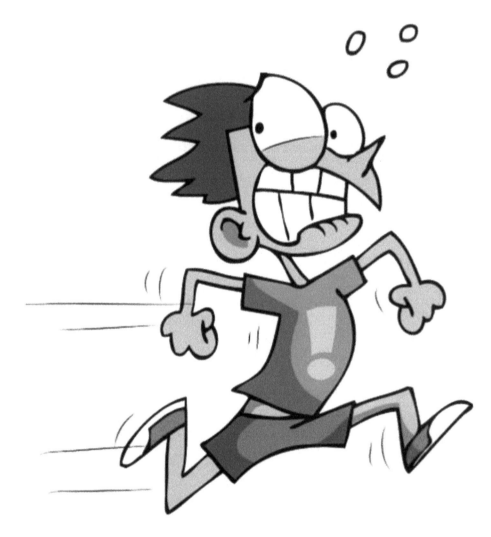

....RUN FOR THE HILLS!!!!!!!

....(you will thank me for it, believe me!)....

….SO HOW LONG DOES IT TAKE TO GROW NEW MUSCLE….

When it comes to muscle growth, you can actually grow more muscle at a quicker rate if you're new to the gym. The longer you've been lifting weights, the longer it takes and the harder it becomes to gain new muscle size.

As a general rule of thumb, you can expect the following when it comes to gaining **new** muscle

NUMBER OF YEARS TRAINING	NEW MUSCLE GAIN (Pounds per Year)	NEW MUSCLE GAIN (Pounds per Month)
1	20-25	2
2	10-12	1
3	5-6	0.5
4	2-3	0.25

Lyle McDonald's Natural Lean Muscle Mass Gains Model

So if you're **new** to the gym, you could gain up to 2 pounds per month naturally (ie. without steroids). If you've been lifting nice and heavy for 3-4 years on a consistent basis, on the other hand, then **new** muscle growth would be significantly less. The point here is that it's easier to build **new** muscle as a beginner as opposed to an experienced weight-lifter or bodybuilder.

....AND HOW LONG DOES IT TAKE TO BURN FAT???....

When it comes to genuine fat loss, you want to ideally **drop your daily calorie-intake by approximately 15% whilst ensuring you've got a decent macronutrient ratio (ie. make sure you're eating enough protein and fat).**

Sure, **you could lose more fat quicker**, but it will be very difficult to sustain. Also if you drop your calorie-intake too much too quickly, you'll probably lose muscle mass too. Believe me, your body won't thank you for it. In fact, the chances are you'll end up losing fat at a slower rate in the long-term for a multitude of reasons beyond the scope of this book.

This is why I would rather you remained **patient yet consistent**.

Since each and every one of us carry **different amounts of fat**,
I would suggest first **assessing your body fat percentage**.

There are many ways by which this can be done such as 'body fat callipers,' 'bod pod,' 'bioelectrical impedance,' 'hydrostatic weighing,' 'dual-energy x-ray absorptiometry (DXA), and 'online calculators.'

Now if you don't want to go through all of that, then you can get a **rough idea** of your body fat percentages by looking at the pictures on the opposite page and seeing where you stand. You can then use the table below that to give you **an idea** about how much weight you should be **aiming** to lose each week.

As a general rule of thumb, **most men will start to look lean at around 10-14% body fat range. Women start to look Jean around the 15-19& body fat range**.

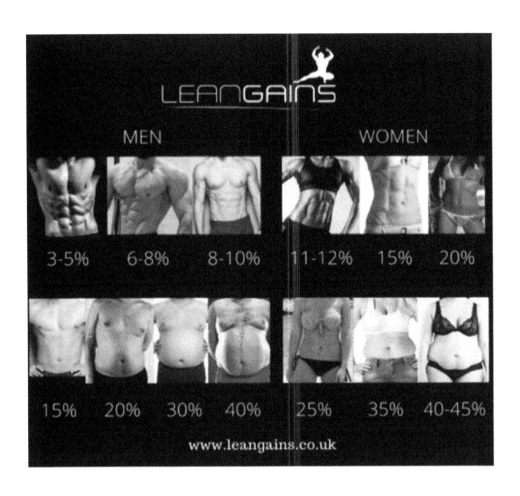

BODY FAT (%)	IDEAL WEIGHT LOSS/WEEK
30+	2lbs/0.9kg
20-30	1.5lbs/0.7-0.9kg
15-20	1.25lbs/0.55-0.7kg
12-15	1-1.25lbs/0.45-0.55kg
9-12	0.75-1lbs/0.35-0.45kg
7-9	0.5-0.75lbs/0.2-0.35kg
7 AND UNDER	0.5lbs/0.2kg

417

..SO, IN CONCLUSION…

You will hopefully realise by now that there really is **no one rule for everybody!** Anybody who tells you that there is…well, chances are they're trying to sell you something. The bottom line here is that some people will make 'lean gains' quicker than others.

The aforementioned calculations give you an idea about how quickly these physical changes can be expected.

To further understand the relevance of these figures and how they relate to both fat-loss and muscle-gain, then I would strongly suggest getting hold of a copy of my other book 'Lean Gains (2nd edition) [if you don't like reading, the 'Lean Gains' book is also available as an audiobook from www.leangains.co.uk].

The first 10 weeks of My 'Lean Gains' Journey!!

So, you can check out my story at **www.leangains.co.uk**, but in a nutshell, it took me **10 months** to drop 18% off my body fat. This **eventually** got me the 6-pack I'd always been yearning for!

However, when I started off, I was clinically obese with a body fat percentage of 28%. I remember feeling desperate to lose the weight as quickly as possible. I also remember how frustrated I felt after 3 weeks of dieting and training and looking exactly the same as I did in the beginning. I never gave up, however, because I understood that in order to be successful, it was important for me to remain consistent. Fat loss and muscle growth are extremely slow processes, and it's always best to take your time and remain patient.

Anyway, for those readers who like to see legitimate before and after pictures, then why not check out the pics on the right. It took me more than 6 months to eventually get the 6-pack, but the pics on page 419 give you an idea of what can be achieved in 10-weeks if you do all the right things.

THE FIRST 10 WEEKS OF MY 'LEAN GAINS' JOURNEY!!

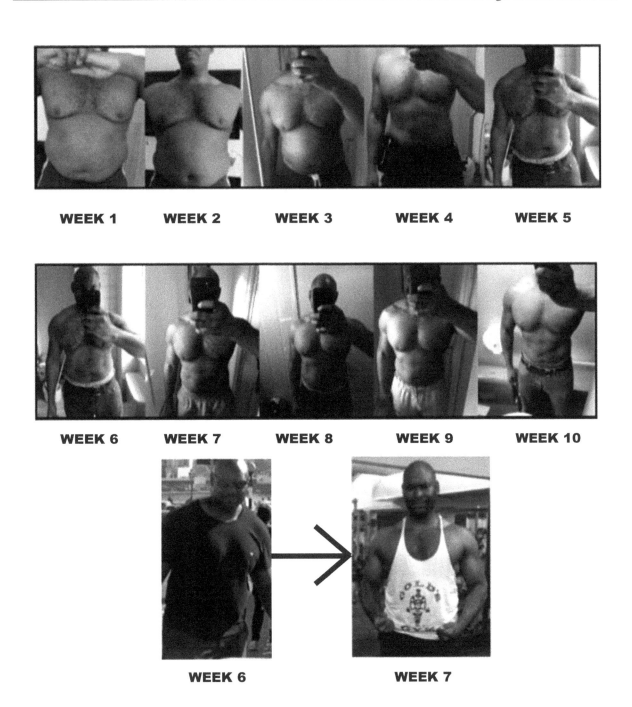

WEEK 1   WEEK 2   WEEK 3   WEEK 4   WEEK 5

WEEK 6   WEEK 7   WEEK 8   WEEK 9   WEEK 10

WEEK 6   WEEK 7

MIKE'S 6-WEEK JOURNEY!!

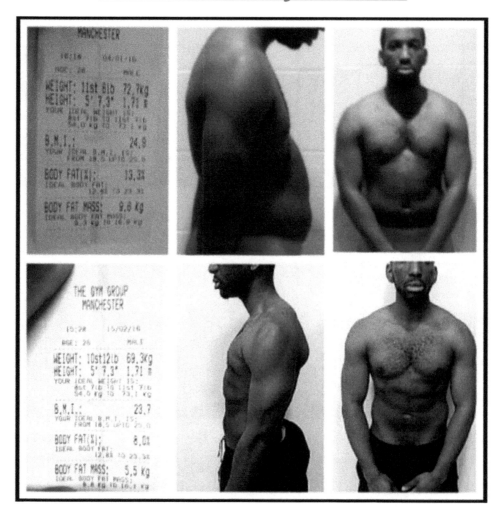

Mike's 6-Week Journey

Another story I like to share is of my friend Mike.
After undertaking the workouts in this book and following
the 'lean gains' diet regimen (check out the book 'How To Get The
Perfect Body'), he managed to lose an incredible 7 pounds in
6 weeks.

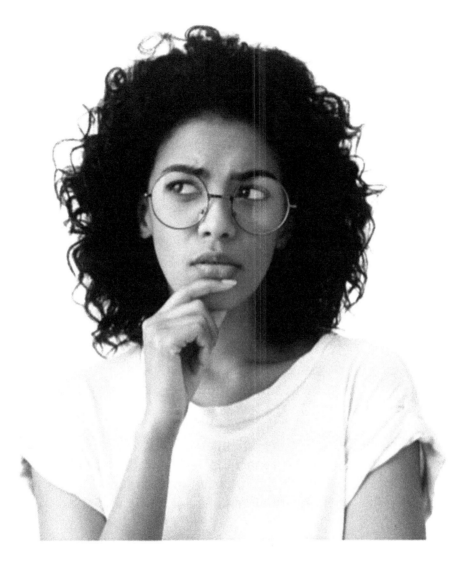

I'M A WOMAN.
WILL LIFTING WEIGHTS
MAKE ME BIG AND BULKY?

....FOR THE LOVE OF GOD, NO!!!!!!....

The commonest reason why **many women** do **not** lift weights is because they're afraid it will make them look butch, 'masculine,' or 'muscular.'

The reality, however, is that this is a **very rare outcome.**

Unless she's in a constant caloric-surplus, has the 'right' genetics and/or makes weight gain an absolute priority, it's unlikely that she will attain a 'bodybuilder' physique.

The beauty of weight training, however, is that it allows you to pretty much attain the body you want (to some degree) if you plan your workouts and diet in advance.

If we take an example of a woman who wants to build a **bigger butt** whilst looking toned and athletic, then she can do so by undergoing the following:

1. Assessing her body fat percentage. If under 18-20%, then the focus should be muscle growth on a 10% calorie-surplus. If over 20%, then the focus should be training on a calorie-deficit of around 15%.

2. Exercises would include hip thrusts, squats and deadlifts as well as accessory workouts such as 'the donkey-kick machine' for instance. Using the suggested exercises within this book as well as progressive overload, her gluteal muscles will get bigger. Over time, this will result in an athletic yet round and shapely appearance.

3. If she's bulking and training for 6 months or so, for instance, then by the end of the 6 months, she would have a bigger butt, but would have also likely accumulated some fat during the bulking process.

4. She can then continue training on a calorie-deficit until she gets back to 18-20% or less. If the sole objective of a female trainee, on the other hand, is to keep the muscle but lose the fat, then she can maintain her muscle yet also strip off the outer layer of fat by doing the following:

1) Assessing her body fat percentage. If she's 30% body fat, for instance, then the focus should be weight training and some cardio on a calorie-deficit.

2) By doing this, she is literally stripping off the body fat without losing muscle.

3) Cardio is optional, but only as a means of accentuating a calorie-deficit and improving overall fitness. In time, she would reach a body fat percentage of 18-20% whilst attaining enough lean muscle to allow for a more shapely appearance as opposed to a skinny/flat appearance, for example.

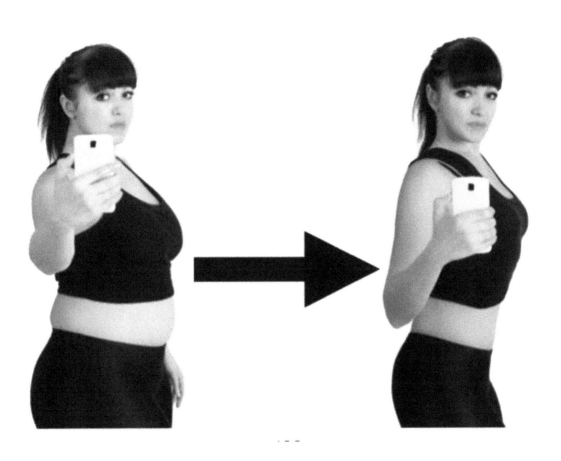

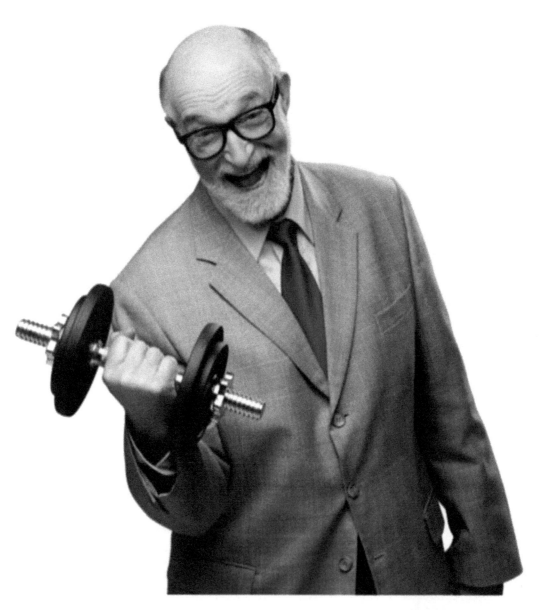

AM I TOO OLD
FOR THIS?

424

….NO!! NOT AT ALL!!….

- From the age of around 30, we naturally lose approximately 3 to 5% muscle mass per decade. This is called **sarcopenia**. In addition, the amount of testosterone we produce starts to decline from the age of 40. This cumulatively results in accelerated muscle loss over the age of 40.

- Common symptoms (both direct and indirect) of sarcopenia include:

- Arthritis

- Reduced Height

- Joint Pain and Physical Disabilities.

- Chronic Inflammation

- Cancer

- Diabetes and Poor Blood Sugar Balance

- Memory Loss

- Weakness

- Depression

- Loss of Independence

- Weight (Fat) Gain

- Sexual Dysfunction

- Poor Circulation

- Reduced Immunity

- Frailty

- The bottom line is that muscle is, and always has been, the **organ of longevity.** This is why so many doctors, personal trainers, nurses, 'fitness gurus', physiotherapists, osteopaths, psychologists, nutritionists, surgeons, dieticians, oncologists and even dentists recommend partaking in at least some form of exercise on a daily basis.

- Now when it comes to exercise and preserving (or even growing) muscle, resistance training is **by far** the best form of exercise.

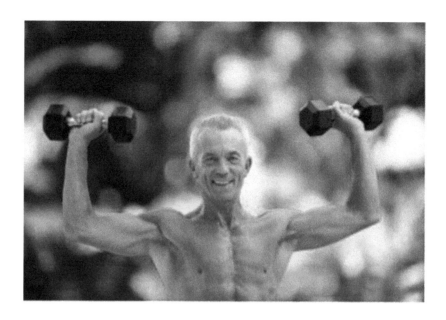

THE GOOD NEWS

- The good news here is that **IT'S NEVER TOO LATE TO GET STARTED!**

- Remember, muscle is the organ of longevity, and weight training has been shown time and again to prevent, significantly slow down and even reverse the symptoms listed above that are often associated with 'old age.'

- But don't take my word for it. There's a ton of research out there that's reached the same conclusion (5,6,33).

- In fact, in one study, 49 participants were split into 2 groups. 1 group consisted of 18-22 year olds and another group consisted 35-50 year olds. They were both puton the same 8 week weight-lifting programme, but the older group gained even more muscle and strength than the younger group.

- Similar results can be seen in people over the age of 60. Studies have demonstrated significant reduction and even reversal of sarcopenia, as well as muscle and strength gains in elderly trainees who have started weight training programmes (6).

THINGS TO LOOK OUT FOR

- We are **more** prone to back pain, arthritis and joint/knee pain as we get older. It's, therefore, prudent to consult your doctor before starting any weight-lifting programme.

- In addition, if you've never done weight lifting before, always start with a light weight in the 10-20 rep range and **perfect** your form before applying progressive overload.

- If you are prone to **arthritis or stiff joints**, lifting super-heavy weights on a regular basis is not a good idea. I would rather you were to follow the advice of your doctor. It's always better, however, to err on the side of caution under such circumstances. Instead of continuously increasing the weight, focus more on gradually increasing your rep range whilst using lighter weights.

- One should also visit his/her physiotherapist on a regular basis to alleviate any 'muscle knots,' aches and pains that may getting the way of blood flow and recovery.

- Another thing to be aware of is that **recovering from a workout will take longer** at the age of 80 as opposed to when you were 18, for example. In other words, it will take longer to recover from a workout as you age, so listen to your body. If your chest is still hurting from the 'pec' session 5 days ago, then wait a few more days before hitting those muscles again.

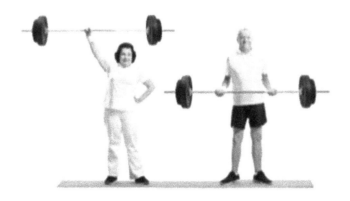

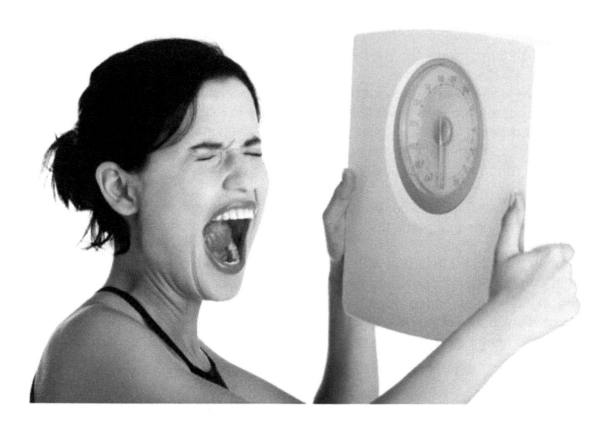

I'VE BEEN DIETING FOR AGES AND CAN'T LOSE WEIGHT!! WHY??

….WELL, LET'S LOOK A BIT

INTO HOW THIS STUFF WORKS…

When you've just began your **weight loss journey** (ie. **once you start eating fewer calories**), you can expect to go through the following 3 phases:

The 3 Phases of Fat Loss

1) <u>Water Loss</u>

- When you start a new eating and exercises regime, you will lose a lot of weight in the beginning.

- This usually occurs during the first couple of weeks, and many people attribute this rapid loss in weight to 'fat.' In reality, most of the weight you lose in the first week or so of dieting will be water-weight. You cannot and will note lose a notable amount of fat in the first week, even if it looks like you are.

2) <u>The 'Adaptation' Phase</u>

- If done correctly, your new 'lifestyle change' will set off a series of hormonal and neurological changes. These changes will optimise, heal and repair many of the internal organs that are involved in converting your body into a 'fatburning machine.'

- Depending on the individual, this may range from a **few days to a month**.

- During this phase, you may **not** see a huge change in your physical appearance, but you will feel stronger, healthier, happier and more vibrant. Your energy levels will increase and you'll start craving more 'healthy foods' and fewer 'unhealthy' foods less.

3) Fat Burning

- Your body likes fat and **doesn't want** to get rid off it right away. This is especially true when it comes to the **stubborn fat** that accumulates around the stomach area (in men) and the hips, butt, and thigh area (in women). In fact, back in the days of the 'hunter-gatherer,' storing loads of fat on your body was a good thing.

- Back then, we didn't know when or where our next meal was coming from. Being 'fat' would keep us alive during the cold, winter months when survival was key.

- Of course nowadays, this isn't a problem for most of us, but our bodies have been conditioned over time to preserve fat wherever and whenever possible. We therefore have to tweak our body's hormonal system a bit so as to instigate and initiate the fat-burning process.

- You can expect **up to 4-6 weeks** before you start to notice a consistent weekly reduction in body fat percentages, and even then, you'll likely hit weight-loss plateaus.

Most dieters don't have a problem losing weight in the beginning.

The real problems often start after a few weeks or months of dieting when further weight loss becomes increasingly difficult.

Once you've been dieting for a while and are maintaining a calorie-deficit, then further weight-loss plateaus are usually due to a drop in **'metabolic rate.'**

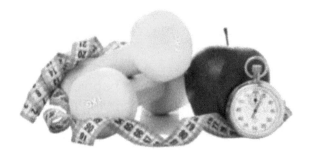

<u>HOW TO REVERSE A</u>
<u>WEIGHT-LOSS PLATEAU</u>

- So you've been dieting for a while, you've been losing weight, and then all of a sudden, despite maintaining a calorie-deficit, you:

  - Stop losing weight,

  - Start craving the 'naughty stuff,'

  - Become tired and lack energy,

  - Start to look and feel weaker than before,

  - Lack energy in the gym!

**When this starts to happen, your body is basically
SCREAMING at you to chill out and take a break!!!**

And that's exactly what you need to do!! That's the cool thing about flexible dieting. It allows you to take a break from your diet for a couple of weeks (this is known as having a 'diet break.'

Basically, **take a break** from the gym every 2 months or so for around 1 week. Don't worry, you won't lose any muscle in a week.

At the same time, take a break from your diet!! This doesn't mean eat pizza and chips all day, but it does mean that you can treat yourself to few extra portions of rice, sweet potato, etc. for a **week or 2**.

When you do this for a couple of weeks, you're essentially:

- Recharging your batteries,
- Increasing your metabolic rate again (which allows you to burn more fat whilst sitting on your sofa).
- Boosting your energy levels (so you can go back to having decent gym sessions).
- Revitalising your body!!

It's a win! win!

Just don't overdo it!!

….Of course, I talk about this in more detail in my other books **'Lean Gains' (2nd Edition) and 'The Essential Guide to Sports Nutrition and Bodybuilding.'**

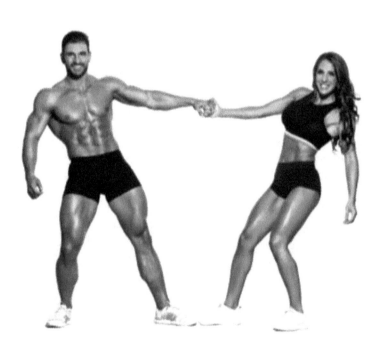

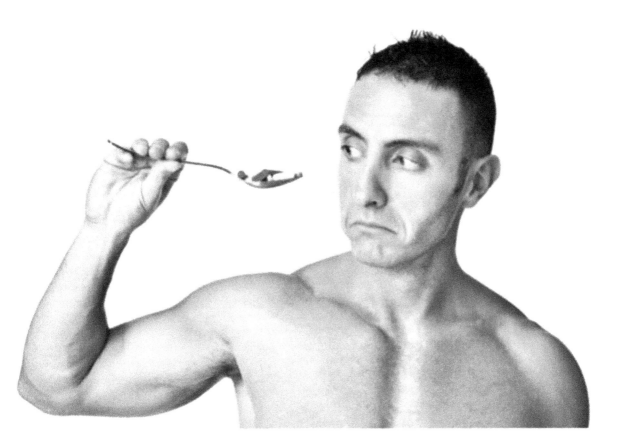

MY FRIENDS IN THE GYM TAKE STEROIDS. SHALL I DO THE SAME?

....WELL, LET'S FIRST LOOK AT WHY STEROIDS ARE SO POPULAR...

What Are Steroids?

- Steroid-drugs are basically man-made versions of naturally-occurring steroid hormones that are made in the body. There are different types of steroid drugs available, but when it comes to exercise and bodybuilding, we're really talking about **'anabolic steroids.'** Anabolic steroids are synthetic substances similar to the male sex hormone 'testosterone.'

- The body cannot differentiate between endogenous (produced naturally by the body) testosterone and the artificial version of it.

What Type of Popular Anabolic Steroids Are Available?

- Androstenedione (Andro)

- Methandrostenolone (Dianabol)

- Oxymetholone (Anadrol-50)

- Testosterone (Sustanon 250, Winstrol)

- Boldenon

- Nandrolone

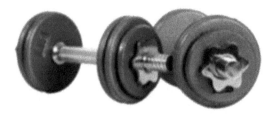

….SO, WHAT WOULD YOU ACHIEVE FROM TAKING THESE DRUGS?…

Significant and Rapid Muscle Growth and Increased Bone Strength

- Well put it this way, a first time steroid user who lifts weights can gain up to 15 pounds in 3 months. Most of this new weight consists **largely** of muscle mass. Compare that to 'natural' gains of up to 1-2 pounds per month, and you can see the appeal. Your bones also become stronger!

Boosts Performance, Strength, and Energy Levels

- Once you start taking this stuff, your energy levels, strength, physical and mental energy will go through the roof. You will feel as like 'The Incredible Hulk' every time you hit the gym.

Improved Determination and Drive

- A surge in testosterone levels increases determination, drive and mental focus.

Reduces Body Fat Levels

- You grow copious amounts of muscle, significantly increase metabolic rate, and become more active when you're on anabolic steroids. This directly and indirectly leads to more fat burning.

Boosts Libido Like Crazy

- Testosterone is the predominant hormone involved in sperm production and the development of male sex organs. It also plays a massive role in sexual arousal and libido. It should come as no surprise, therefore, that your sexdrive will go through the roof once you start taking anabolic steroids.

...SOUNDS GOOD SO FAR!
WHAT'S THE PROBLEM???..

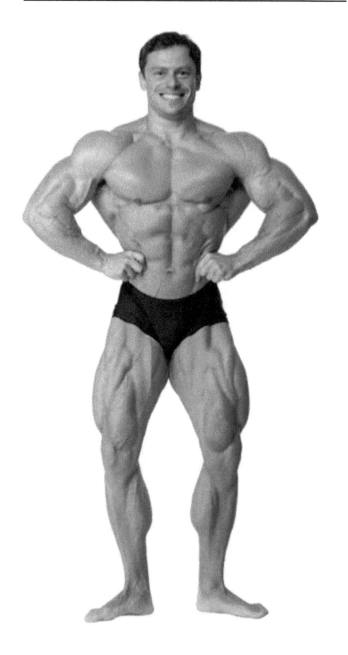

....WELL, IT'S NOT ALL FINE AND DANDY. THERE ARE SOME DOWNSIDES TOO...

Higher Risk of Heart Failure, Atherosclerosis, and Cancer

- Prolonged steroid-use has been linked to a variety of cardiovascular and heart problems. Examples include cardiomyopathy, heart-failure, and atherosclerosis. This can lead to death in some long-term steroid users.

- Prolonged steroid use has been linked to liver cancer and liver adenomas in many users.

Unpredictable Changes in Behaviour

- You may have heard of the dreaded 'roid-rage' in some users. However, in reality, behaviour and mood changes associated with steroid-use are diverse and un-preditable. They can range from severe aggression to euphoria.

Shrinking Gonads (Balls)

- When you take steroids, you're introducing loads more testosterone to the body than the amount you produce naturally. This adversely affects your hormonal balance meaning you produce less natural testosterone. Since a lot of testosterone is made in the testicles (balls), they will shrink because they become less active.

Acne and Hair Loss

- You have a 50% chance of developing severe acne once you start taking this stuff. There have also been many links to baldness.

...SO, SHOULD YOU TAKE STEROIDS OR NOT?..

What I Have Seen For Myself

- I have never taken steroids before, and don't see myself doing so. I have, how ever, personally trained with 5 people in my life who are taking/have taken steroids. 2 of those trainees were long-term users with whom I had been training for almost a year. I won't use their real names because they didn't want me to, but let's call them Pete and Andy.

- The physical changes I noticed in just 6 months of training with them were truly unbelievable. I mean they packed on a noticeable amount of muscle in such an incredibly short time period.

- But what surprised me the most was how quickly they were able to recover after a heavy weight training session. It would take me at least a few days to recover after a hard-and-heavy chest day, yet these 2 guys could have easily done another intense chest workout the very next day if they wanted to.

- Their energy levels were much higher than mine, and they were able to progress much quicker than me when it came to adding plates to the bar and progressive overload on the whole. Sure, I was progressing too, but by no means as quickly as Pete and Andy. I would often talk to them about sex and libido. They both told me that they would often feel 'more horny' during the day, and were able to have sex more frequently than usual. In fact, Pete would often tell me about how he would have sex with his girlfriend 5 times a day when he first started taking steroids (which I think is quite a lot). When it came to side effects, Andy did notice a shrinkage in the size of his balls, but Pete apparently didn't. In the beginning, they both experienced some acne, but this disappeared after a month or so.

- I must admit, when I was training with Pete and Andy, I was tempted to take steroids myself, especially after seeing how quickly they packed on new muscle.

- Pete and Andy still take steroids to this very day with few (if any) real side effects. Most people who take steroids do so in 'cycles.' This is what Pete and Andy did. At the beginning of a cycle, they would start with a low dose and then slowly increase the doses. In the second half of the cycle, the doses are slowly decreased to zero. There are times when they would continue to train for a few weeks without taking any steroids and then go back on them. In fact, most steroid users believe that doing these cycles allows the body time to adjust to the high doses, and the drug-free cycle allows the body's hormonal system time to recuperate.

- Now this all seems fine and dandy, but my main deterrent was always, and still is, the long-term side effects. Remember I said that I've trained with five people in my life who take, or have taken, steroids? Well, one of those five trainees passed away recently due to heart failure. Although I did not know this guy that well, he apparently had no previous medical conditions, but he was taking some form of anabolic steroids for over ten years.

- And then there are the multitude of bodybuilders on steroids who have passed away as a result of some form of associated heart problem or multi-organ failure. Famous examples include Dallas McCarver, Andreas Münzer, Mike Matarazzo, Greg Kovacs, Rich Piana, Dan Puckett, and the list goes on.

- So, am I saying that taking anabolic steroids will kill you or shorten your life eventually? Well, possibly. I know there are people like Pete and Andy who absolutely swear by it. I honestly do not see them going back to a life without steroids, and I can understand that. I mean think about it, you are no longer producing a significant amount of testerone naturally anymore since your body is operating on this synthesised version. Despite all the wonderful and amazing effects of this drug, the fact remains that you're no longer producing a normal level of natural testosterone because of this.

- So what's going to happen when you stop taking it?? You're going to feel like crap! You will feel weak, you'll have no sex drive, you'll lack strength and energy, and feel extremely depressed. This is especially the case if your body's already dependent on it. Of course, this won't last forever, and you will likely start producing normal amounts of testosterone again, but this won't compare to the copious amount you were injecting into yourself every day. So this really beckons the question, 'why take it in the first place?'

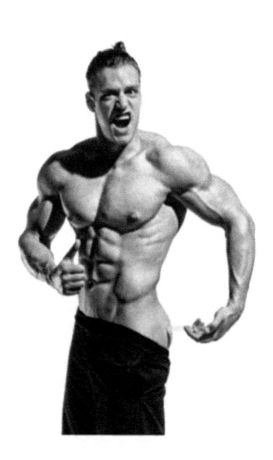

...SO, WHAT'S THE CONCLUSION..

"No matter how great the talent or efforts, some things just take time. You can't produce a baby in one month by getting nine women pregnant."

Warren Buffett

- Some things just take time. Muscle growth is a slow process for most of us. Sure, there are some trainees out there who can grow a copious amount of muscle at a quicker rate than others, and the reasons why boil down to genetics to some degree. However, for those out there who find it difficult to burn fat or build muscle (hard-gainers), the temptation to accelerate the process is mighty tempting.

- I would never judge anyone who decides to go down the 'steroid' route and I totally understand the appeal. The results that I've seen first hand are truly incredible.

- However, it may be difficult for some users to stop after seeing such incredible results, not to mention the enhanced sex drive, strength, physical appearance, etc.

- The questions you have to ask yourself are 'Am I going to do this forever?' and 'If I keep it up, am I willing to put up with the adverse sideeffects linked to long-term use?'

- The bottom line is that you can make incredible 'lean gains' without resorting to juicing up your muscles. Once you apply the tried-andtested science behind it to your diet and your workouts, you WILL without doubt achieve some amazing results, live a long and healthy life, and look and feel great **without** resorting to any drugs at all! The only downside with doing this naturally is that it will take longer....so there you have it, the choice is yours at the end of the day.

...AND THAT'S ALL FOLKS!!..

"Thank you so much for taking time out to read this book. I sincerely hope you find the principles covered throughout to be useful, and I wish you the very best moving forwards."

Dr Jonathan S. Lee

THE 'LEAN GAINS' BOOK COLLECTION

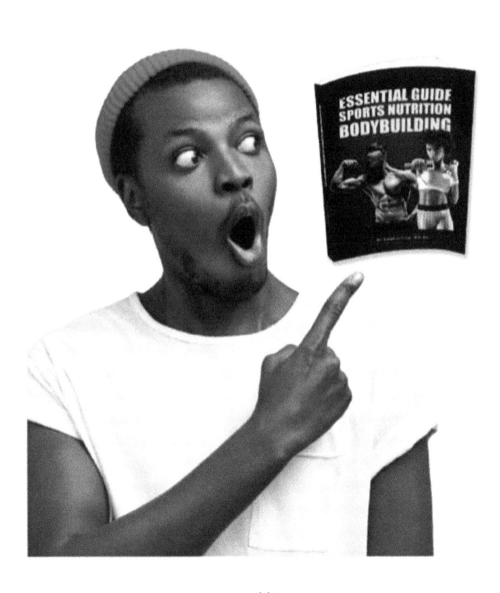

THE ESSENTIAL GUIDE TO SPORTS NUTRITION AND BODYBUILDING

'**The Essential Guide to Sports Nutrition and Bodybuilding**' contains **everything** you need to know about losing weight, eating right, gaining muscle, feeling great, and living a long, healthy, and vibrant life.

Outstanding Features include:

- **800 pages** of attractive, easy-to-digest information covering a huge range of topics.

- **Science-backed information** and advice based on over **580 clinical studies and references**.

- Over **254 full-colour photographs** and illustrations.

- Simple descriptions, paragraph breaks, and a **key-point summary** at the end of each chapter to allow for enjoyable reading.

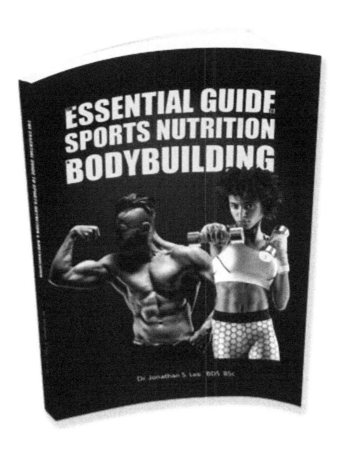

LEAN GAINS
(2nd Edition)

'Lean Gains (2nd edition)' is an absolute MUST for those who are struggling to burn fat, bulk up, and break through weight-loss plateaus. Dr Lee has created a comprehensive blueprint to help manage your weight and achieve faster results than you would using conventional dieting methods.

Outstanding Features include:

- **470 pages** of easy-to-digest information relating to the science behind fat-loss and muscle gain.

- **Science-backed information** and advice based on over **500 clinical studies and references.**

- Over **200 full-colour photographs** and illustrations.

- **Paragraph breaks**, colour pictures on almost every page, and a gentle sense of humour for enjoyable reading.

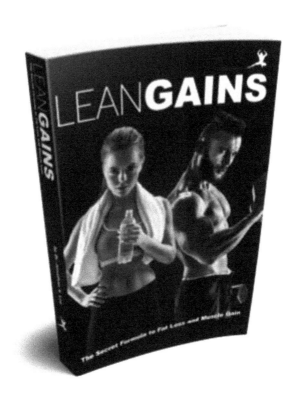

HARDBACK:	£49.99
PAPERBACK:	£45.99
EBOOK:	£9.99
AUDIOBOOK:	£9.99

(prices may vary)

AVAILABLE AT

WWW.LEANGAINS.CO.UK

and

Amazon

THE ULTIMATE GYM WORKOUT

'**The Ultimate Gym Workout**' is the perfect adjunct to your gym workouts. This book sets in place a series of effective, tried-and-tested gym workouts. Designated set ranges, rep ranges, rest periods, and stretching routines take away the need to focus on anything other than the workouts themselves.

Outstanding Features include:

- **155 full-colour photographs and illustrations.**

- Detailed **weight-training** and **cardio workouts.**

- Simple descriptions and video links (ebook version).

- **Exercise routines** tailored for both **men and women.**

- **Stretching routines** tailored for both **men and women.**

- Choice between **3-day and 5-day workouts.**

- All exercises are **fully explained** and **illustrated**.

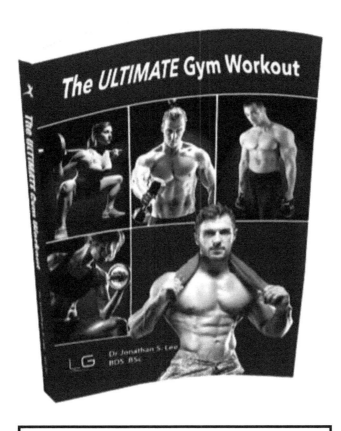

HARDBACK:	N/A
PAPERBACK:	£44.99
EBOOK:	£9.99

(prices may vary)

AVAILABLE AT

WWW.LEANGAINS.CO.UK

and

Amazon

YOUR POCKETBOOK GUIDE TO THE ULTIMATE GYM WORKOUT

'Your Pocketbook Guide to The Ultimate Gym Workout' is the 'pocketbook' accompaniment to its larger parent book **'The Ultimate Gym Workout.'**

This book sets in place a series of effective tried-and-tested gym workouts.

Outstanding Features include:

• Detailed **weight-training** and **cardio workouts.**

• Simple descriptions and video links (ebook version).

• **Exercise routines** tailored for both **men and women.**

• Choice between **3-day and 5-day workouts.**

• All exercises are **fully explained** and **illustrated.**

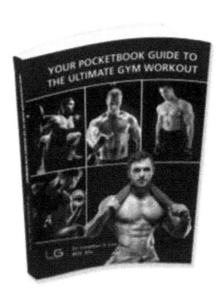

HOW TO GET THE PERFECT BODY

'How to Get The Perfect Body' is a no-BS introduction
to the world of diet and fitness.

'How To Get The Perfect Body'
is extremely easy on the eye, contains a plethora
of paragraph breaks, images, before & after pictures, and
can be read from front to back in less than an hour.

However, this book contains **calculations and formulae**,

used by most fitness models and bodybuilders, that you

will not find in most fitness books.

By the time you've finished reading this book, you
will know exactly how to achieve that **sexy** body you've
been craving for all this time

No exercise routines are contained within this book.

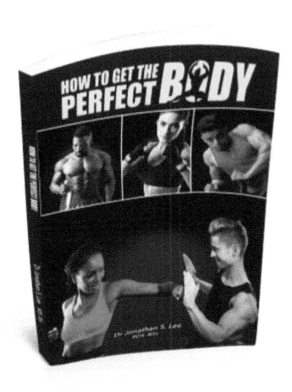

HARDBACK:	**£19.99**
PAPERBACK:	**£14.99**
EBOOK:	**£9.99**

(prices may vary)

AVAILABLE AT

WWW.LEANGAINS.CO.UK

and

Amazon

LEAN MEALS
FOR EVERYONE

Eating regimes and dieting habits vary massively from one person to the next. Some dieters, for instance, prefer a ketogenic approach, whilst others may prefer to go vegan.

Some trainees prefer a calorie-based eating regime, whilst others feel more comfortable fasting for prolonged periods of time. The point is that one set of fixed meal plans is very unlikely to cater for everyone.

Dr Lee wrote **'Lean Meals for Everyone'** as a means of addressing these issues.

This book contains a wide range of healthy and nutritious recipes and meal plans that will suit specific caloric and nutritional requirements regardless of diet.

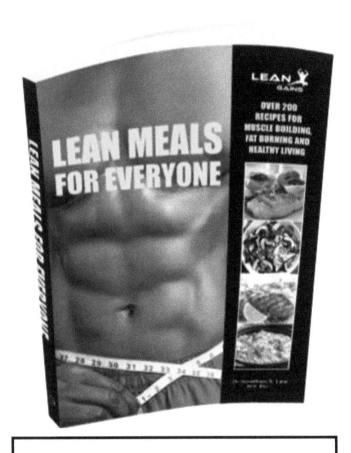

HARDBACK:	N/A
PAPERBACK:	£29.99
EBOOK:	£9.99

(prices may vary)

AVAILABLE AT

WWW.LEANGAINS.CO.UK

and

Amazon

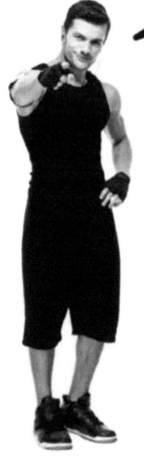

YOUR FEEDBACK IS IMPORTANT TO US!

If you like what you've read, then please take a minute to write a few words on Amazon about this book. I check all my reviews and love to receive feedback.

If you have any queries, questions, or concerns about anything, on the other hand, then please feel free to drop me an email at

jon@leangains.co.uk

and we will try our best to resolve your issue.

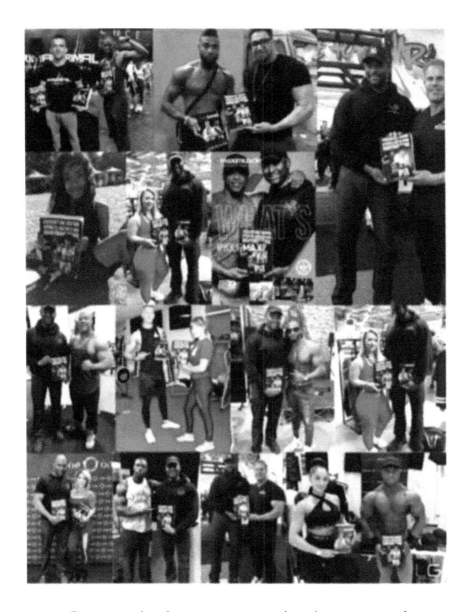

For more books, events, merchandise, personal trainers, fitness professionals, testimonials, viodes, blogs and upcoming events, then please visit www.leangains.co.uk

REFERENCES

BOOKS

Aragon A. (2007) Girth Control: *The Science of Fat Loss and Muscle Gain, 1st Edition.*

Bean A. **The Complete Guide to Strength Training 5th edition**

Contreras B. (2013) *Bodyweight Strength Training Anatomy*

Delavier F. (2010) *Strength Training Anatomy, 3rd Edition.*

Delavier F. (2011) *Delavier's Core Training Anatomy.*

Gleeson, M. and Maughan R. (2004) *The Biochemical Basis of Sports Performance, New York: Oxford University Press Inc.*

Hinson J, Raven P and Chew S. (2010) *The Endocrine System, 2nd Edition, London: Churchill Livingstone Elsevier.*

Hofmekler O. (2008) *Maximum Muscle, Minimum Fat,* Berkeley, California: North Atlantic Books.

MacLaren D. and Morton J. (2012) *Biochemistry for Sport and Exercise Metabolism,* West Sussex: Blackwell Publishing.

Jay (2017) *Superior Fat Loss.* Available Online (e-book). AworkoutRoutine.com

Jay (2017) *Superior Muscle Growth.* Available Online (e-book). AworkoutRoutine.com

Lee J (2018) *The Essential Guide to Sports Nutrition and Bodybuilding.* Available Online. www.leangains.co.uk

Lee J (2018) *Lean Gains (Second Edition).* Available Online. www.leangains.co.uk

McDonald L. (1998) *The Ketogenic Diet: A Complete Guide for The Dieter and Practitioner,* 1st Edition, Austin Tx: Lyle McDonald Publishing.

McDonald L. (2005) *A Guide to Flexible Dieting: How Being Less Strict With Your Diet Can Make It Work Better,* 1st Edition, Salt Lake City.

McDonald L. (2008) *The Rapid Fat Loss Handbook: A Scientific Approach to Crash Dieting,* 2nd Edition, Salt Lake City: Lyle McDonald Publishing.

McDonald L. (2003) *The Ultimate Diet 2.0: Advanced Cyclical Dieting for Achieving Super Leanness,* 1st Edition, Salt Lake City: Lyle McDonald Publishing.

McDonald L. and Helms E. (2018) *The Women's Book: Vol 1; A Guide to Nutrition, Fat Loss and Muscle Gain*: Lyle McDonald Publishing.

Matthews M. (2014) *Bigger, Leaner, Stronger,* 2nd Edition, USA: Oculus Publishers.

Matthews M. (2016) *The Shredded Chef: 120 Recipes for Building Muscle, Getting Lean, and Staying Healthy,* USA: Andrea Lynn, et al.

Salway J. G. (2004) *Metabolism at a Glance , 3rd Edition,* Oxford: Blackwell Publishing Ltd.

REFERENCES

PAPERS

1. Kelleher AR, Hackney KJ, Fairchild TJ, Keslacy S, Ploutz-Snyder LL. "The metabolic costs of reciprocal supersets vs. traditional resistance exercise in young recreationally active adults." *J Strength Cond Res. 2010 Apr;24(4):1043-51*. Available at: https://www.ncbi.nlm.nih.gov/pubmed/20300020

2. Horowitz JF, Mora-Rodriguez R, Byerley LO, Coyle EF. "Lipolytic suppression following carbohydrate ingestion limits fat oxidation during exercise." *Am J Physiol. 1997 Oct;273(4 Pt 1):E768-75*. Available at: https://www.ncbi.nlm.nih.gov/pubmed/9357807

3. Willardson JM. "A brief review: factors affecting the length of the rest interval between resistance exercise sets." *J Strength Cond Res. 2006 Nov;20(4):978-84*. Available at: https://www.ncbi.nlm.nih.gov/pubmed/17194236

4. Iglay HB, et al. "Resistance training and dietary protein: effects on glucose tolerance and contents of skeletal muscle insulin signaling proteins in older persons." *Am J Clin Nutr. 2007 Apr;85(4):1005-13*. Available at: https://www.ncbi.nlm.nih.gov/pubmed/17413099

5. Evans WJ. "Reversing sarcopenia: how weight training can build strength and vitality." *Geriatrics. 1996 May;51(5):46-7, 51-3*. Available at: https://www.ncbi.nlm.nih.gov/pubmed/8621102

6. Marini M, Sarchielli E, Brogi L, Lazzeri R, Salerno R, Sgambati E, Monaci M. "Role of adapted physical activity to prevent the adverse effects of the sarcopenia. A pilot study." *Ital J Anat Embryol. 2008 Oct-Dec;113(4):217-25*. Available at: https://www.ncbi.nlm.nih.gov/pubmed/19507462

7. Stronger by Science. "Sex Differences in Training and Metabolism" January 2015. Available at: https://www.strongerbyscience.com/gender-differences-in-training-and-diet/

8. Cory T. Walts et al. "Do Sex or Race Differences Influence Strength Training Effects on Muscle or Fat?" *Med Sci Sports Exerc. 2008 Apr; 40(4): 669–676*. Available at:https://www.ncbi.nlm.nih.gov/pmc/articles/PMC2991130/

9. Gibala, M, et al. "Metabolic adaptations to short-term high-intensity interval training: A little pain for a lot of gain?" *Exercise and Sports Sci Rev 2008;36:58-63*.

10. Brad Schoenfeld. "Bro-Split Versus Total-Body Training: Which Builds More Muscle?" http://www.lookgreatnaked.com/blog/bro-split-versus-total-body-training-which-builds-more-muscle/

11. Kerksick, Chad M et al. "Early-Phase Adaptations to a Split-Body, Linear Periodization Resistance Training Program in College Aged and Middle-Aged Men" *The Journal of Strength & Conditioning Research: May 2009 - Volume 23 - Issue 3 - p 962-971*. Available online at: https://journals.lww.com/nsca-jscr/Fulltext/2009/05000/Early_Phase_Adaptations_to_a_Split_Body,_Linear.35.aspx

REFERENCES

12. Radaelli R, Fleck SJ, Leite T, Leite RD, Pinto RS, Fernandes L, Simão R. "Dose-response of 1, 3, and 5 sets of resistance exercise on strength, local muscular endurance, and hypertrophy." *J Strength Cond Res. 2015 May;29(5):1349-58* Available at: https://www.ncbi.nlm.nih.gov/pubmed/25546444

13. Amirthalingam T, Mavros Y, Wilson GC, Clarke JL, Mitchell L, Hackett DA. "Effects of a Modified German Volume Training Program on Muscular Hypertrophy and Strength." *J Strength Cond Res. 2017 Nov;31(11):3109-3119.*

14. Schoenfeld BJ, Ratamess NA, Peterson MD, Contreras B, Sonmez GT, Alvar BA. "Effects of different volume-equated resistance training loading strategies on muscular adaptations in well-trained men." *J Strength Cond Res. 2014 Oct;28(10):2909-18.* Available at https://www.ncbi.nlm.nih.gov/pubmed/24714538

15. Shepstone TN, Tang JE, Dallaire S, Schuenke MD, Staron RS, Phillips SM. "Short-term high- vs. low-velocity isokinetic lengthening training results in greater hypertrophy of the elbow flexors in young men." *J Appl Physiol (1985). 2005 May;98(5):1768-76.* Available at:https://www.ncbi.nlm.nih.gov/pubmed/15640387

16. Fitts RH, McDonald KS, Schluter JM. "The determinants of skeletal muscle force and power: their adaptability with changes in activity pattern." *J Biomech. 1991;24 Suppl 1:111-22.* Available at:https://www.ncbi.nlm.nih.gov/pubmed/1791172

17. Mujika, Padilla S. "Scientific bases for pre-competition tapering strategies." *J Med Sci Sports Exerc. 2003 Jul;35(7):1182-7.* Available at:https://www.ncbi.nlm.nih.gov/pubmed/12840640

18. Kazunori Nosaka, Priscilla M. ClarksonMary E. McGuigginJames M. Byrne "Time course of muscle adaptation after high force eccentric exercise." *European Journal of Applied Physiology and Occupational Physiology 1991, Vol 63, Issue 1, pp70-76.* Available Online at: https://link.springer.com/article/10.1007/BF00760804

19. de Salles BF, Simão R, Miranda F, Novaes Jda S, Lemos A, Willardson JM. "Rest interval between sets in strength training." *Sports Med. 2009;39(9):765-77.* Available Online at: https://www.ncbi.nlm.nih.gov/pubmed/19691365

20. Rosenkilde, M, et al. "Body fat loss and compensatory mechanisms in response to different doses of aerobic exercise--a randomized, controlled trial in overweight, sedentary males." *Am J Physiol Regul Integr Comp Physiol 2012;303;R573=R579.*

21. Fisher, JP, et al. "The effects of pre-exhaustion, exercise order, and rest intervals in a full-body resistance training intervention." *Appl Physiol Nutr Matab 2014.*

22. Sousa, M, et al. "Dietary strategies to recover from exercise-induced muscle damage." Int J Food Sci Nutr 2103.

23. Wernbom M, Augustsson J, Thomeé R. "The influence of frequency, intensity, volume and mode of strength training on whole muscle cross-sectional area in humans." Sports Med. 2007;37(3):225-64

24. Schoenfeld BJ, Peterson MD, Ogborn D, Contreras B, Sonmez GT. "Effects of Low- vs. High-Load Resistance Training on Muscle Strength and Hypertrophy in Well-Trained Men" *J Strength Cond Res. 2015 Oct;29(10):2954-63*

25. Gerald T Mangine, Jay R Hoffman, Adam M Gonzalez, Jeremy R Townsend, Adam J Wells, Adam R Jajtner, Kyle S Beyer, Carleigh H Boone, Amelia A Miramonti, Ran Wang, Michael B LaMonica, David H Fukuda, Nicholas A Ratamess and Jeffrey R Stout. "The effect of training volume and intensity on improvements in muscular strength and size in resistance-trained men." *Physiol Rep. 2015 Aug; 3(8): e12472* Available at: https://www.ncbi.nlm.nih.gov/pmc/articles/PMC4562558/

REFERENCES

26. Mangine GT et al. "Resistance training intensity and volume affect changes in rate of force development in resistance-trained men." *Eur J Appl Physiol. 2016 Dec;116(11-12):2367-2374*

27. McGuigan MR, Newton MJ, Winchester JB, Nelson AG. "Relationship between isometric and dynamic strength in recreationally trained men." *J Strength Cond Res. 2010 Sep;24(9):2570-3.*

28. Sanmy R. Nóbrega and Cleiton A. Libardi. "Is Resistance Training to Muscular Failure Necessary?" *Front Physiol. 2016; 7: 10*

29. Burke LM, Hawley JA, Ross ML, Moore DR, Phillips SM, Slater GR, Stellingwerff T, Tipton KD, Garnham AP, Coffey VG. "Preexercise aminoacidemia and muscle protein synthesis after resistance exercise." Med Sci Sports Exerc. 2012 Oct;44(10):1968-77 Schoenfeld BJ, Peterson MD, Ogborn D, Contreras B, Sonmez GT. "Effects of Low- vs. High-Load Resistance Training on Muscle Strength and Hypertrophy in Well-Trained Men" *J Strength Cond Res. 2015 Oct;29(10):2954-63*

30. Gerald T Mangine, Jay R Hoffman, Adam M Gonzalez, Jeremy R Townsend, Adam J Wells, Adam R Jajtner, Kyle S Beyer, Carleigh H Boone, Amelia A Miramonti, Ran Wang, Michael B LaMonica, David H Fukuda, Nicholas A Ratamess and Jeffrey R Stout. "The effect of training volume and intensity on improvements in muscular strength and size in resistance-trained men." *Physiol Rep. 2015 Aug; 3(8): e12472* Available at: https://www.ncbi.nlm.nih.gov/pmc/articles/PMC4562558/

31. Mangine GT et al. "Resistance training intensity and volume affect changes in rate of force development in resistance-trained men." *Eur J Appl Physiol. 2016 Dec;116(11-12):2367-2374*

32. McGuigan MR, Newton MJ, Winchester JB, Nelson AG. "Relationship between isometric and dynamic strength in recreationally trained men." *J Strength Cond Res. 2010 Sep;24(9):2570-3.*

33. Law TD, Clark LA, Clark BC. "Resistance Exercise to Prevent and Manage Sarcopenia and Dynapenia." *Annu Rev Gerontol Geriatr. 2016; 36(1): 205–228.*

PICTURES
Original (Non-Stock) Photos

1. Lee S. " Flat Barbell Bench Press; Starting Position Jamie." Energie Fitness - Chelmsley Wood. *Native Pixel.*

2. Lee S. " Flat Barbell Bench Press; Finishing Position Jamie." Energie Fitness - Chelmsley Wood. *Native Pixel.*

3. Lee S. " Inclined Barbell Bench Press; Starting Position of Jamie." Energie Fitness - Chelmsley Wood. *Native Pixel.*

4. Lee S. " Inclined Barbell Bench Press; Finishing Position of Jamie." Energie Fitness - Chelmsley Wood.*Native Pixel.*

5. Lee S. "Inclined Dumbbell Bench Press; Starting Position of Jamie." Energie Fitness - Chelmsley Wood. *Native Pixel.*

6. Lee S. "Inclined Dumbbell Bench Press; Finishing Position of Jamie." Energie Fitness - Chelmsley Wood.. *Native Pixel.*

REFERENCES

7. Lee S. "Dumbbell Pullover; Starting Position of Jamie." Energie Fitness - Chelmsley Wood.. *Native Pixel.*

8. Lee S. "Dumbbell Pullover; Finishing Position of Jamie." Energie Fitness - Chelmsley Wood.. *Native Pixel.*

9. Lee S. "Dumbbell Flyes; Starting Position of Dermot Gallagher." Genesis Gym, London. *Native Pixel.*

10. Lee S. "Dumbbell Flyes; Finishing Position of Dermott Gallagher." Genesis Gym, London. *Native Pixel.*

11. Lee S. "Cable Crossover-Upper; Starting Position of Chris Halgreen." Solihull College Gym, Solihull. *Native Pixel.*

12. Lee S. "Cable Crossover-Upper; Finishing Position of Chris Halgreen." Solihull College Gym, Solihull. *Native Pixel.*

13. Lee S. "Dips; Starting Position of Molly" Simply Gym, Walsall. *Native Pixel.*

14. Lee S. "Dips; Finishing Position of Molly" Simply Gym, Walsall. *Native Pixel.*

15. Lee S. "Overhead Press; Chris Halgreen" Solihull College Gym, Solihull. *Native Pixel.*

16. Lee S. " Military Press; Starting Position Jamie." Energie Fitness - Chelmsley Wood. *Native Pixel.*

17. Lee S. " Military Press; Finishing Position Jamie." Energie Fitness - Chelmsley Wood. *Native Pixel.*

18. Lee S. "Arnold-Press; Starting Position of Chris Halgreen." Solihull College Gym, Solihull. *Native Pixel.*

19. Lee S. "Arnold-Press; Finishing Position of Chris Halgreen." Solihull College Gym, Solihull. *Native Pixel.*

20. Lee S. "Dumbbell Raise; Starting Position of Chris Halgreen." Solihull College Gym, Solihull. *Native Pixel.*

21. Lee S. "Dumbbell Raise; Finishing Position of Chris Halgreen." Solihull College Gym, Solihull. *Native Pixel.*

22. Lee S. "Overhand Grip for Chris Halgreen." Solihull College Gym, Solihull. *Native Pixel.*

23. Lee S. "Dumbbell Front Raise; Starting Position of Chris Halgreen." Solihull College Gym, Solihull. *Native Pixel.*

24. Lee S. "Dumbbell Front Raise; Starting Position of Chris Halgreen." Solihull College Gym, Solihull. *Native Pixel.*

25. Lee S. "Dumbbell Front Raise; Starting Position of Molly" Simply Gym, Walsall. *Native Pixel.*

26. Lee S. "Dumbbell Front Raise; Finishing Position of Molly" Simply Gym, Walsall. *Native Pixel.*

27. Lee S. "Seated Rear Delt Raise; Starting Position of Chris Halgreen." Solihull College Gym, Solihull. *Native Pixel.*

28. Lee S. "Seated Rear Delt Raise; Finishing Position of Chris Halgreen." Solihull College Gym, Solihull. *Native Pixel.*

29. Lee S. "Lyndsey: The Clean Grip." Solihull College Gym, Solihull. *Native Pixel.*

30. Lee S. "Barbell Front Squat; Starting Position." Simply Gym, Walsall. *Native Pixel.*

31. Lee S. "Barbell Front Squat; Finishing Position." Simply Gym, Walsall. *Native Pixel.*

REFERENCES

32. Lee S. "Romanian Deadlift; Starting Position of Chris Halgreen." Solihull College Gym, Solihull. *Native Pixel.*

33. Lee S. "Romanian Deadlift; Finishing Position of Chris Halgreen." Solihull College Gym, Solihull. *Native Pixel.*

34. Lee S. "Barbell Calf Raise; Starting Position of Chris Halgreen." Solihull College Gym, Solihull. *Native Pixel.*

35. Lee S. "Barbell Calf Raise; Finishing Position of Chris Halgreen." Solihull College Gym, Solihull. *Native Pixel.*

36. Lee S. "Barbell Calf Raise; Starting Position of Dermot Gallagher." Genesis Gym, London. *Native Pixel.*

37. Lee S. "Barbell Calf Raise; Finishing Position of Dermot Gallagher." Genesis Gym, London. *Native Pixel.*

38. Lee S. "Seated Calf Raise; Starting Position of Dermot Gallagher." Genesis Gym, London. *Native Pixel.*

39. Lee S. "Seated Calf Raise; Finishing Position of Dermot Gallagher." Genesis Gym, London. *Native Pixel.*

40. Lee S. "Calf Raise on Leg Press; Starting Position of Dermot Gallagher." Genesis Gym, London. *Native Pixel.*

41. Lee S. "Calf Raise on Leg Press; Finishing Position of Dermot Gallagher." Genesis Gym, London. *Native Pixel.*

42. Lee S. "Barbell Bicep Curl; Starting Position of Chris Halgreen." Solihull College Gym, Solihull. *Native Pixel.*

43. Lee S. "Barbell Bicep Curl; Finishing Position of Chris Halgreen." Solihull College Gym, Solihull. *Native Pixel.*

44. Lee S. "Barbell E-Z Bicep Curl; Starting Position of Chris Halgreen." Solihull College Gym, Solihull. *Native Pixel.*

45. Lee S. "Barbell E-Z Bicep Curl; Finishing Position of Chris Halgreen." Solihull College Gym, Solihull. *Native Pixel.*

46. Lee S. "Hammer Curl; Starting Position of Chris Halgreen." Solihull College Gym, Solihull. *Native Pixel.*

47. Lee S. "Hammer Curl; Finishing Position of Chris Halgreen." Solihull College Gym, Solihull. *Native Pixel.*

48. Lee S. "Chin-up; Starting Position of Chris Halgreen." Solihull College Gym, Solihull. *Native Pixel.*

49. Lee S. "Chin-up Finishing Position of Chris Halgreen." Solihull College Gym, Solihull. *Native Pixel.*

50. Lee S. "Close-Grip Barbell Press; Starting Position of Jamie." Energie Fitness - Chelmsley Wood. *Native Pixel.*

51. Lee S. "Close-Grip Barbell Press; Finishing Position of Jamie." Energie Fitness - Chelmsley Wood.. *Native Pixel.*

52. Lee S. "Dips; Starting Position of Jamie." Energie Fitness - Chelmsley Wood. *Native Pixel.*

53. Lee S. "Dips; Finishing Position of Jamie." Energie Fitness - Chelmsley Wood.*Native Pixel.*

54. Lee S. "Skull-Crushers; Starting Position of Jamie." Energie Fitness - Chelmsley Wood. *Native Pixel.*

55. Lee S. "Skull-Crushers; Finishing Position of Jamie." Energie Fitness - Chelmsley Wood. *Native Pixel.*

REFERENCES

56. Lee S. "Skull-Crushers; Starting Position of Chris Halgreen." Solihull College Gym, Solihull. *Native Pixel.*

57. Lee S. "Skull-Crushers; Finishing Position of Chris Halgreen." Solihull College Gym, Solihull. *Native Pixel.*

58. Lee S. "Dumbbell Overhead Tricep Press; Starting Position of Chris Halgreen." Solihull College Gym, Solihull. *Native Pixel.*

59. Lee S. "Dumbbell Overhead Tricep Press; Finishing Position of Chris Halgreen." Solihull College Gym, Solihull. *Native Pixel.*

60. Lee S. "Dumbbell Overhead Tricep Press; Starting Position of Jamie." Energie Fitness - Chelmsley Wood.*Native Pixel.*

61. Lee S. "Dumbbell Overhead Tricep Press; Finishing Position of Jamie." Energie Fitness - Chelmsley Wood.*Native Pixel.*

62. Lee S. "Tricep Pushdown; Starting Position of Chris Halgreen." Solihull College Gym, Solihull. *Native Pixel.*

63. Lee S. "Tricep Pushdown; Finishing Position of Chris Halgreen." Solihull College Gym, Solihull. *Native Pixel.*

64. Lee S. "Barbell Deadlift Overgrip; Chris Halgreen." Solihull College Gym, Solihull. *Native Pixel.*

65. Lee S. "Barbell Deadlift Mixed grip; Chris Halgreen." Solihull College Gym, Solihull. *Native Pixel.*

66. Lee S. "Barbell Deadlift; Starting Position of Chris Halgreen." Solihull College Gym, Solihull. *Native Pixel.*

67. Lee S. "Barbell Deadlift; Finishing Position of Chris Halgreen." Solihull College Gym, Solihull. *Native Pixel.*

68. Lee S. "Wide-Grip; Starting Position of Chris Halgreen." Solihull College Gym, Solihull. *Native Pixel.*

69. Lee S. "Wide-Grip; Finishing Position of Chris Halgreen." Solihull College Gym, Solihull. *Native Pixel.*

70. Lee S. "Wide-Grip; Starting Position of Dermot Gallagher." Genesis Gym, London. *Native Pixel.*

71. Lee S. "Wide-Grip; Finishing Position of Dermot Gallagher." Genesis Gym, London. *Native Pixel.*

72. Lee S. "Hyperextension; Starting Position of Molly" Simply Gym, Walsall. *Native Pixel.*

73. Lee S. "Hyperextension; Finishing Position of Molly" Simply Gym, Walsall. *Native Pixel.*

74. Lee S. "Bar Attached to Pulley" Simply Gym, Walsall. *Native Pixel.*

75. Lee S. "Hanging Straight Leg Raise; Starting Position of Chris Halgreen." Solihull College Gym, Solihull. *Native Pixel.*

76. Lee S. "Hanging Straight Leg Raise; Finishing Position of Chris Halgreen." Solihull College Gym, Solihull. *Native Pixel.*

77. Lee S. "Captain Chair Knee Raise; Starting Position of Molly (Front and Side)" Simply Gym, Walsall. Native Pixel.

78. Lee S. "Captain Chair Knee Raise; Finishing Position of Molly (Front and Side)" Simply Gym, Walsall. *Native Pixel.*

79. Lee S. "Captain Chair Straight Leg Raise; Starting Position of Molly (Front and Side)" Simply Gym, Walsall. *Native Pixel.*

REFERENCES

80. Lee S. "Captain Chair Straight Leg Raise; Finishing Position of Molly (Front and Side)" Simply Gym, Walsall. *Native Pixel.*

81. Lee S. "Decline Sit-Up; Starting Position of Molly" Simply Gym, Walsall. *Native Pixel.*

82. Lee S. "Decline Sit-Up; Starting Position of Molly" Simply Gym, Walsall. *Native Pixel.*

83. Lee S. "Hip Thrusts; Starting Position of Jamie." Energie Fitness - Chelmsley Wood. *Native Pixel.*

84. Lee S. "Hip Thrusts; Finishing Position of Jamie." Energie Fitness - Chelmsley Wood.*Native Pixel.*

85. Lee S. "Bulgarian Split Squat; Starting Position of Molly" Simply Gym, Walsall. *Native Pixel.*

86. Lee S. "Bulgarian Split Squat; Finishing Position of Molly" Simply Gym, Walsall. *Native Pixel.*

87. Lee S. "Donkey-Kick Machine Close Up of Molly's Feet" Simply Gym, Walsall. *Native Pixel.*

88. Lee S. "Donkey-Kick Machine; Starting Position of Molly" Simply Gym, Walsall. *Native Pixel.*

89. Lee S. "Donkey-Kick Machine; Finishing Position of Molly" Simply Gym, Walsall. *Native Pixel.*

90. Lee S. "Facepull; Starting Position of Chris Halgreen." Solihull College Gym, Solihull. *Native Pixel.*

91. Lee S. "Facepull; Finishing Position of Chris Halgreen." Solihull College Gym, Solihull. *Native Pixel.*

92. Lee S. "Dumbbell Internal Rotation; Starting Position of Chris Halgreen." Solihull College Gym, Solihull. *Native Pixel.*

93. Lee S. "Dumbbell Internal Rotation; Finishing Position of Chris Halgreen." Solihull College Gym, Solihull. *Native Pixel.*

94. Lee S. "Dumbbell External Rotation; Starting Position of Chris Halgreen." Solihull College Gym, Solihull. *Native Pixel.*

95. Lee S. "Dumbbell External Rotation; Finishing Position of Chris Halgreen." Solihull College Gym, Solihull. *Native Pixel.*

Stock Photos

1. https://www.shutterstock.com/image-photo/fit-woman-stretching-her-leg-warm-107519378?src=library&studio=1

2. https://www.shutterstock.com/image-photo/attractive-woman-exercising-wheel-roller-abs-485228521?src=library&studio=1

3. https://www.shutterstock.com/image-photo/attractive-woman-exercising-wheel-roller-abs-485228527?src=library&studio=1

4. https://www.shutterstock.com/image-photo/closeup-picture-hanging-handle-machine-gym-682778617?src=library&studio=1

5. https://www.shutterstock.com/image-photo/young-handsome-fit-man-performing-backextension-1062808007?src=library&studio=1

REFERENCES

6. https://www.shutterstock.com/image-photo/young-handsome-fit-man-performing-backextension-1040623021? src=library&studio=1

7. https://www.shutterstock.com/image-photo/muscular-man-workout-gym-doing-exercises-1407145670?src=library&studio=1

8. https://www.shutterstock.com/image-photo/bodybuilder-working-on-his-chest-cable-407210491?src=library&studio=1

9. https://www.shutterstock.com/image-photo/muscular-men-exercising-weights-he-performing-199554692?src=library&studio=1

10. https://www.shutterstock.com/image-photo/fitness-asian-woman-working-out-shoulder-599406365?src=library&studio=1

11. https://www.shutterstock.com/image-photo/shoulder-pull-down-machine-fitness-man-1027353787?src=library&studio=1

12. https://www.shutterstock.com/image-photo/girl-gym-crouches-barbell-beautiful-sports-1087014974?src=library&studio=1

13. https://www.shutterstock.com/image-photo/girl-gym-crouches-barbell-beautiful-sports-1087014974?src=library&studio=1

14. https://www.shutterstock.com/image-photo/girl-gym-crouches-barbell-beautiful-sports-1087014977?src=library&studio=1

15. https://www.shutterstock.com/image-photo/athlete-doing-pullup-on-horizontal-barmans-218472940?src=library&studio=1

16. https://www.shutterstock.com/image-photo/male-powerlifter-starting-deadlift-barbell-gym-1226590138?src=library&studio=1

17. https://www.shutterstock.com/image-photo/closeup-muscular-man-doing-deadlift-exercise-519486769?src=library&studio=1

18. https://www.shutterstock.com/image-illustration/french-press-barbell-lying-3d-illustration-419748157?src=library&studio=1

19. https://www.shutterstock.com/image-photo/young-bodybuilder-training-gym-triceps-close-69079699?src=library&studio=1

20. https://www.shutterstock.com/image-illustration/decline-bench-282776015?src=library&studio=1

21. https://www.shutterstock.com/image-photo/fit-young-woman-doing-bicycle-crunch-1026889825?src=library

22. https://www.shutterstock.com/image-photo/side-view-young-woman-doing-situps-776994154?src=library

23. https://www.shutterstock.com/image-photo/muscular-male-doing-crossfit-training-749638846?src=library

24. https://www.shutterstock.com/image-photo/fit-couple-going-practice-yoga-against-89051245?src=library

25. https://www.shutterstock.com/image-photo/bicep-curl-exercise-studio-shot-over-314080721?src=library&studio=1

26. https://www.shutterstock.com/image-photo/hammer-curl-exercise-studio-composite-over-373995424?src=library&studio=1

27. https://www.shutterstock.com/image-photo/personal-trainer-doing-standing-dumbbell-curls-139687066?src=library&studio=1

28. https://www.shutterstock.com/image-illustration/dumbbell-biceps-curl-3d-illustration-622379480?src=library&studio=1

REFERENCES

29. https://www.shutterstock.com/image-illustration/curl-dumbbell-grip-3d-illustration-428906812?src=library&studio=1

30. https://www.shutterstock.com/image-illustration/curls-barbell-undergrip-3d-illustration-421075573?src=library&studio=1

31. https://www.shutterstock.com/image-photo/beautiful-fitness-young-sporty-couple-dumbbell-202116130?src=library&studio=1

32. https://www.shutterstock.com/image-photo/gym-interior-standing-calf-raises-machine-176115239?src=library&studio=1

33. https://www.shutterstock.com/image-illustration/smith-machine-282776027?src=library&studio=1

34. https://www.shutterstock.com/image-illustration/standing-calf-raises-3d-illustration-434632420?src=library&studio=1

35. https://www.shutterstock.com/image-photo/young-man-doing-seated-bent-over-263444261?src=library&studio=1

36. https://www.shutterstock.com/image-photo/fitness-girl-sportswear-doing-deadlift-exercise-1301900572?src=library&studio=1

37. https://www.shutterstock.com/image-vector/sport-exercise-physical-training-right-wrong-568197397?src=library&studio=1

38. https://www.shutterstock.com/image-photo/muscular-men-lifting-deadlift-gym-1084435391?src=library&studio=1

39. https://www.shutterstock.com/image-photo/barbell-lunges-360744425?src=library&studio=1

40. https://www.shutterstock.com/image-photo/beautiful-fitness-woman-working-out-studio-200273168?src=library&studio=1

41. https://www.shutterstock.com/image-photo/fitness-sport-bodybuilding-exercising-people-concept-795968392? src=library&studio=1

42. https://www.shutterstock.com/image-photo/fitness-sport-bodybuilding-exercising-people-concept-625131833? src=library&studio=1

43. https://www.shutterstock.com/image-photo/weightlifter-getting-ready-stand-heavy-barbell-1014369187?src=library&studio=1

44. https://www.shutterstock.com/image-photo/man-doing-back-squat-exercise-raising-623720516?src=library&studio=1

45. https://www.shutterstock.com/image-photo/weight-lifter-lifting-weights-during-competition-264171473?src=library&studio=1

46. https://www.shutterstock.com/image-photo/two-strong-men-gym-sport-335648897?src=library&studio=1

47. https://www.shutterstock.com/image-photo/handsome-weightlifter-lifting-bench-press-working-1135133126?src=library&studio=1

48. https://www.shutterstock.com/image-photo/dumbbell-pull-over-exercise-studio-shot-474551074?src=library&studio=1

49. https://www.shutterstock.com/image-illustration/dumbbell-bench-press-lying-second-embodiment-428906839? src=library&studio=1

50. https://www.shutterstock.com/image-photo/young-bodybuilder-training-gym-chest-barbell-68880256?src=library&studio=1

51. https://www.shutterstock.com/image-photo/muscular-man-lifting-barbell-on-bench-276291302?src=library&studio=1

52. https://www.shutterstock.com/image-photo/grip-barbell-bench-press-276900341?src=library&studio=1

REFERENCES

53. https://www.shutterstock.com/image-photo/muscular-man-doing-heavy-exercise-athletic-357979883?src=library&studio=1

54. https://www.shutterstock.com/image-photo/brutal-athletic-man-pumping-muscles-on-767581144?src=library&studio=1

55. https://www.shutterstock.com/image-photo/young-man-gym-exercising-chest-on-391826842?src=library&studio=1

56. https://www.shutterstock.com/image-photo/beautiful-girl-sports-hall-carries-out-116182342?src=library&studio=1

57. https://www.shutterstock.com/image-photo/fitness-woman-doing-jump-step-ups-1155383425?src=library&studio=1

58. https://www.shutterstock.com/image-photo/beautiful-young-woman-measuring-tape-isolated-116440234?src=library&studio=1

59. https://www.shutterstock.com/image-photo/powerful-bodybuilder-doing-exercises-dumbbells-photo-1289910055? src=library&studio=1

60. https://www.shutterstock.com/image-photo/powerful-bodybuilder-doing-exercises-dumbbells-photo-1289910055? src=library&studio=1

61. https://www.shutterstock.com/image-photo/young-man-shirtless-ball-pointing-you-1298789737?src=library&studio=1

62. https://www.shutterstock.com/image-photo/sports-wall-horizontal-bar-isolated-on-372716224?src=library&studio=1

63. https://www.shutterstock.com/image-photo/muscular-athletic-bodybuilder-fitness-model-posing-478420210?src=library&studio=1

64. https://www.shutterstock.com/image-photo/sport-fitness-barbell-closeup-ez-curl-770596432?src=library&studio=1

65. https://www.shutterstock.com/image-photo/sad-woman-on-diet-vegetables-isolated-76854916?src=library&studio=1

66. https://www.shutterstock.com/image-photo/wheel-abdominal-muscles-ab-workout-fitness-722507113?src=library&studio=1

67. https://www.shutterstock.com/image-illustration/rod-narrow-grip-bench-press-lying-425668651?src=library&studio=1

68. https://www.shutterstock.com/image-photo/technique-doing-exercise-deadlift-barbell-young-658073911?src=library&studio=1

69. https://www.shutterstock.com/image-photo/athletic-young-woman-works-out-pink-126757655?src=library&studio=1

70. https://www.shutterstock.com/image-photo/man-lying-enjoying-on-sandy-tropical-1069679981?src=library&studio=1

71. https://www.shutterstock.com/image-photo/muscular-shirtless-black-male-bodybuilder-drinking-1136212946?src=library&studio=1

72. https://www.shutterstock.com/image-photo/woman-working-out-weights-smile-on-115329358?src=library&studio=1

73. https://www.shutterstock.com/image-photo/muscular-bodybuilder-guy-doing-exercises-dumbbells-176406695? src=library&studio=1

74. https://www.shutterstock.com/image-photo/black-bodybuilder-posing-round-discs-strong-159614729?src=library&studio=1

75. https://www.shutterstock.com/image-photo/beautiful-sporty-muscular-woman-working-out-338402264?src=library&studio=1

REFERENCES

76. https://www.shutterstock.com/image-photo/young-woman-bench-pressing-dumbbells-gym-187286432?src=library&studio=1

77. https://www.shutterstock.com/image-photo/female-bodybuilder-exercising-barbell-isolated-on-248442529?src=library&studio=1

78. https://www.shutterstock.com/image-photo/beautiful-afro-american-sports-girl-working-471992953?src=library&studio=1

79. https://www.shutterstock.com/image-photo/bodybuilder-bodybuilding-muscles-strong-muscular-young-516086359?src=library&studio=1

80. https://www.shutterstock.com/image-illustration/3d-rendering-start-end-position-bulgarian-613219172?src=library&studio=1

81. https://www.shutterstock.com/image-illustration/knee-raise-on-parallel-bars-3d-418402327?src=library&studio=1

82. https://www.shutterstock.com/image-illustration/curling-body-via-block-simulator-3d-418402330?src=library&studio=1

83. https://www.shutterstock.com/image-illustration/hyperextension-3d-illustration-417842911?src=library&studio=1

84. https://www.shutterstock.com/image-illustration/shrugs-dumbbells-3d-illustration-428906824?src=library&studio=1

85. https://www.shutterstock.com/image-illustration/lever-tbar-row-plate-loaded-3d-622379585?src=library&studio=1

86. https://www.shutterstock.com/image-photo/exercise-back-photo-strong-attractive-woman-619943012?src=library&studio=1

87. https://www.shutterstock.com/image-illustration/thrust-rod-standing-slope-3d-illustration-421075636?src=library&studio=1

88. https://www.shutterstock.com/image-photo/young-bodybuilder-resting-between-exercises-isolated-748940587?src=library&studio=1

89. https://www.shutterstock.com/image-photo/muscular-male-dumbbell-isolated-on-white-596464403?src=library&studio=1

90. https://www.shutterstock.com/image-photo/bodybuilder-posing-handsome-power-athletic-guy-259874381?src=library&studio=1

91. https://www.shutterstock.com/image-photo/textbooks-background-73887280?src=library&studio=1

92. https://www.shutterstock.com/image-illustration/rise-on-toes-soleus-simulator-3d-418630501?src=library&studio=1

93. https://www.shutterstock.com/image-photo/man-bodybuilder-white-toque-blanche-cook-334340810?src=library&studio=1

94. https://www.shutterstock.com/image-photo/healthy-hispanic-woman-dumbbells-working-out-114168691?src=library&studio=1

95. https://www.shutterstock.com/image-photo/woman-doing-exercises-abdominal-muscles-isolated-85094836?src=library&studio=1

96. https://www.shutterstock.com/image-photo/sporty-woman-does-exercises-dumbbells-on-642069538?src=library&studio=1

97. https://www.shutterstock.com/image-illustration/3d-illustration-two-chrome-dumbbells-over-93221173?src=library&studio=1

98. https://www.shutterstock.com/image-photo/fitness-sporty-sexy-long-hair-girl-397055857?src=library&studio=1

REFERENCES

99. https://www.shutterstock.com/image-photo/young-happy-woman-isolated-on-white-164262947?src=library&studio=1

100. https://www.shutterstock.com/image-photo/health-fitness-concept-before-after-weight-228979996?src=library&studio=1

101. https://www.shutterstock.com/image-photo/black-bodybuilder-training-dumbbells-strong-man-149726210?src=library&studio=1

102. https://www.shutterstock.com/image-photo/black-bodybuilder-posing-round-discs-strong-149745953?src=library&studio=1

103. https://www.shutterstock.com/image-photo/attractive-athletic-girl-showing-biceps-269789696?src=library&studio=1

104. https://www.shutterstock.com/image-photo/barbell-isolated-on-white-background-1139066726?src=library&studio=1

105. https://www.shutterstock.com/image-illustration/french-press-barbell-lying-3d-illustration-419748157?src=library&studio=1

106. https://www.shutterstock.com/image-photo/confident-black-bodybuilder-smiling-strong-man-151400435?src=library&studio=1

107. https://www.shutterstock.com/image-photo/fit-man-woman-smiling-camera-together-256179067?src=library&studio=1

108. https://www.shutterstock.com/image-photo/muscular-man-doing-exercises-dumbbells-biceps-588411014?src=library&studio=1

109. https://www.shutterstock.com/image-photo/resting-time-sporty-girl-bottle-water-281327639?src=library&studio=1

110. https://www.shutterstock.com/image-photo/beautiful-strong-woman-doing-fitness-plank-618438887?src=library&studio=1

111. https://www.shutterstock.com/image-photo/woman-measuring-leg-hip-measurement-tape-200142854?src=library&studio=1

112. picshutter

113. https://www.shutterstock.com/image-photo/collection-cabbages-isolated-on-white-background-92432269?src=library&studio=1

114. https://www.shutterstock.com/image-photo/nutritionist-saying-no-cake-woman-isolated-167303564?src=library&studio=1

115. https://www.shutterstock.com/image-photo/young-male-athlete-holding-bottle-protein-329808695?src=library&studio=1

116. https://www.shutterstock.com/image-photo/hyderabadi-chicken-dum-biryani-served-kadhai-678254116?src=library&studio=1

117. https://www.shutterstock.com/image-photo/cheerful-muscular-man-standing-healthy-food-243688870?src=library&studio=1

118. https://www.shutterstock.com/image-photo/woman-baggy-pants-thumbs-isolated-over-101421856?src=library&studio=1

119. https://www.shutterstock.com/image-photo/woman-measuring-leg-hip-measurement-tape-200142854?src=library&studio=1

120. https://www.shutterstock.com/image-photo/caprese-salad-on-white-background-410810617?src=library&studio=1

REFERENCES

INTERNET SITES

1. *Muscularstrength.com*
2. *bodybuilding.com*
3. *Athlean-x.com*
4. *wikihow.com*
5. *T-nation.com*
6. *leangains.co.uk*
7. *muscleforlife.com*
8. *www.aworkoutroutine.com*
9. *www.catalystathletics.com/*
10. *exercise.com*

INDEX

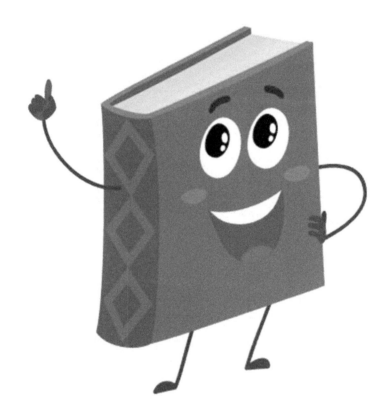

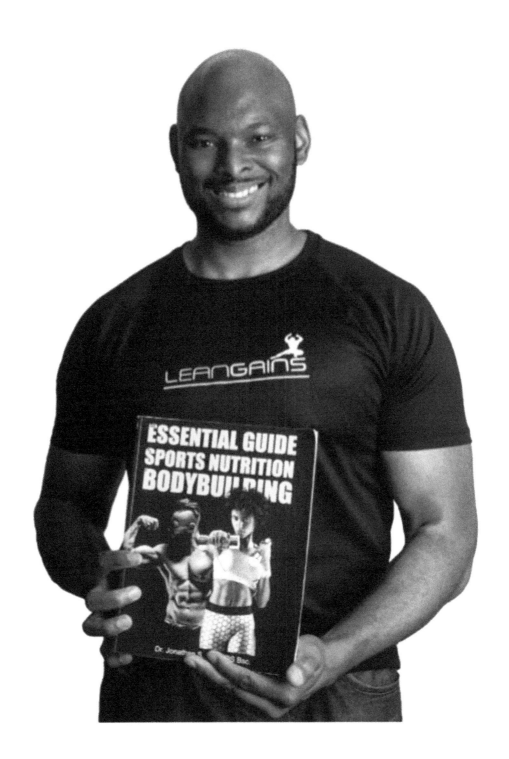

Milton Keynes UK
Ingram Content Group UK Ltd.
UKHW051402020923
427819UK00002B/4